THE DARE

THE DARE

*Can You Walk Away from
Your Poisonous Passion?*

TONY GONZALEZ

Library of Congress Control Number: 2012918833
ISBN: Hardcover   978-1-4797-3011-7
               Softcover   978-1-4797-3010-0
               Ebook   978-1-4797-3012-4

Project Editor: Mike Sigalas

Book Cover Illustration by Tim Kasa

This book was printed in the United States of America.

Rev. date: 05/06/2013

To order additional copies of this book, contact:
Xlibris Corporation
1-888-795-4274
www.Xlibris.com
Orders@Xlibris.com
103833

CONTENTS

This book is dedicated my beautiful wife, who has always been the calming spirit to my temperamental personality. I love you!

It also is dedicated to my children, who serve as constant reminders of the love that God has for me, His child. I love all of you!

And lastly and most importantly, this book is dedicated to God, without whom none of this would have been possible. May all honors that come to me go to Him!

Acknowledgements

I'm grateful to the many people who have been so supportive of me while putting this book together. From those who offered their testimonials, to those who took part in my experiments, throughout the countless revisions and editions, there are many along the way who kept me moving forward through their help, their service, or simply an encouraging word. From the bottom of my heart, thank you!

A special thanks to Bob and Joyce Gonzalez, my parents, for their time and input throughout all of the editing process. I could not have completed this book without them.

I also want to thank all those who allowed me the use of their quotes, statistics, and information. Not being a medical doctor, I had to lean on your wisdom and credibility for the information in this book. Thank you.

To my kids, for cheering me on and giving up time with me so I could work on the book. I think they all deserve one big, tasty, treat—sugar free of course!

Lastly, I want to thank my wife. Katie. This was a five year effort and took a lot of time away from her. They say that behind every great man there is a loving and supporting wife. I believe it. My wife is the perfect woman for me, building me up when I'm low and sharing the highs with me. She supports me even when she could be kicking me in the pants. Katie, I love you and am blessed to be married to you!

Back in October, my husband and I decided to give up sugar (along with white flour and fried foods). We committed to a month . . . not thinking that it would be a long-term decision but would help us to gain better control over our eating habits in the future. The month was not a huge challenge. Eating this new way was easy at home, since we did it together and I do enjoy healthy food too. Going out to eat or to a friend's house for dinner was a bigger challenge simply because more tempting food was around. However, we didn't cheat. During this month, we felt energetic and our minds where "crisper." I loved the feeling of having all the energy and mental capacity I needed to do all of my daily tasks, and though my body didn't look very different, it felt different . . . again, more energetic. I was also more engaged with my family since I had more energy. After that month, my favorite desserts were extra yummy now that I hadn't had sweets in so long; they were much more enjoyable. As the month ended, our goal was to learn from the past month and eat these "treat" foods only on rare occasions; however, these tempting foods quickly made their way into our daily diet. Immediately, my energy level decreased and my mind became more fuzzy. My mood was not as good. It was a very noticeable change. There is a very clear link between what I eat and how my body (and mind) operates.

Kristin
Duluth, GA

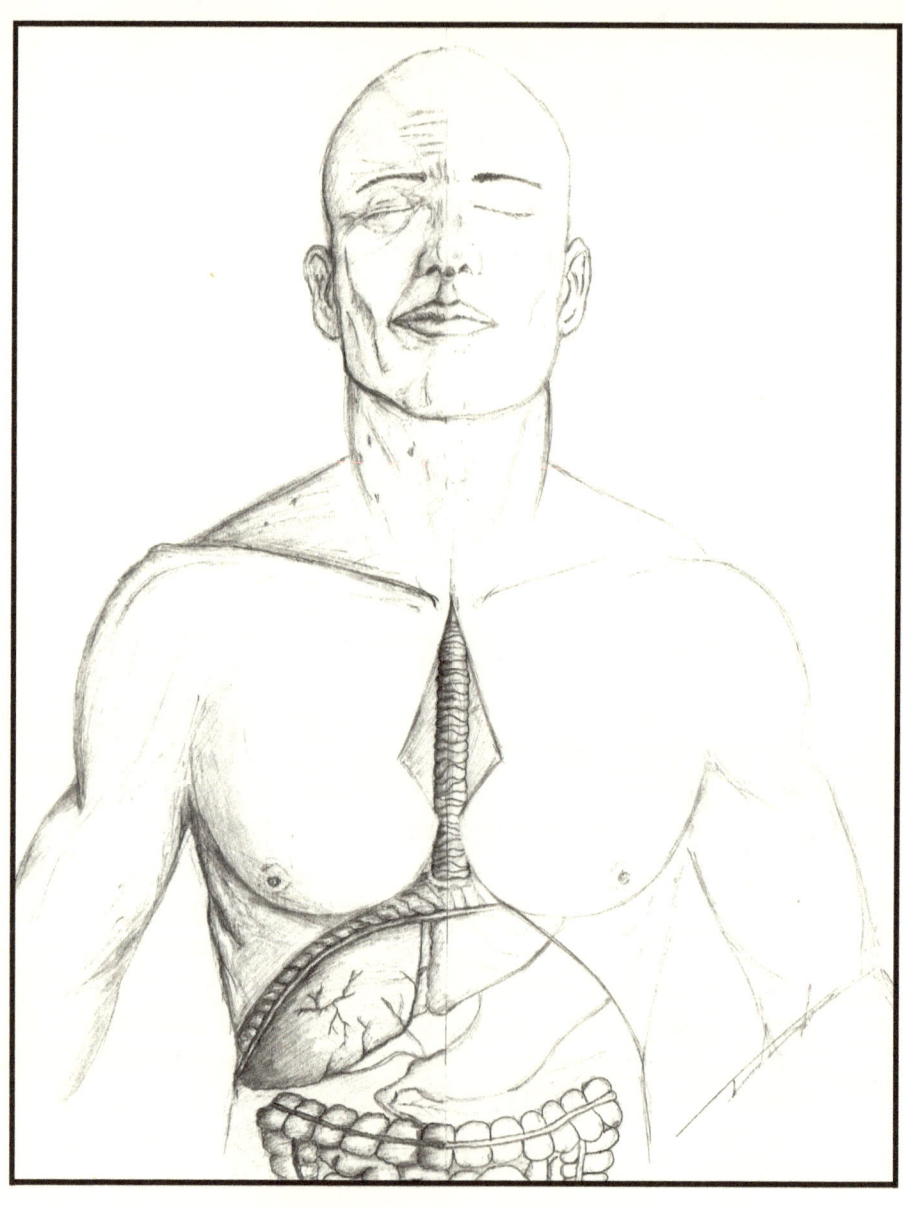

Illustration 1: a man divided, showing the results of the daily choices we make. Remember when your momma told you that you are what you eat? Your cells reproduce themselves over and over so much so that you basically have a new body every seven or so years. So it is literally true, you become what you give your body to reproduce itself!

Chapter 1: Intro to The Dare

Let me guess . . . you have picked this book up because the title was a bit catchy? *No?* Maybe you are interested in living a healthier lifestyle, or maybe you have recently been told by your doctor that you are diabetic and need to watch the sugars in your diet. Maybe you are a parent seeking alternatives to feed your children so they won't keep bouncing off the walls like human pinball machines.

Well, whatever your reason, don't put this book down!

I repeat, don't put this book down!

Instead, read it. It will change your life . . . if you are ready. In this book, I have attempted to take the simple but very important and sensitive topic of "refined sugar in diets" and have put it into terms that anyone can understand. My hopes are that everyone who reads this book will, at a minimum, say, "Wow, I've never really thought about this before; I guess I should."

My goals for this book are threefold:

1. To show you how your digestive system should work and how a healthy body functions
2. To show you how refined sugars are negatively affecting your body and how it is also affecting us as a society at large
3. To provide the needed tools and resources to cut refined sugars from your diet

Along with this, I also want to personally challenge you to what I am calling *The Dare*. I am challenging you to live thirty days without eating refined sugars. It might be something you decide to do for yourself or maybe with your spouse, child, or entire family. But to help you accept this challenge and to succeed in its completion, I've included all of the tools you will need. Shopping list, recipes, a daily schedule . . . it is all there to help you on this new journey.

I'll also be discussing common questions and concerns throughout as well as providing you with better eating tips and personal stories from those who have already taken *The Dare* and who have discovered the benefits of removing the poison that is refined sugar from their diet.

**

About eight years ago, I was forced to remove sugar from my diet. I say *forced* because the only other option was to continue getting sicker. I was suffering at the time from a set of symptoms without a specific name — fatigue, depression, weight loss, unclear thinking, irrational thinking, irritability, and shakiness. I was getting rashes on my hands, feet, elbows, and knees, especially in cold weather. It got so bad that I didn't want to go out much in the wintertime. I was throwing up for no good reason but always feeling better after I did.

I was only thirty-one but beginning to feel like my body was breaking down and that my quality of life was fading. I was married at the time, with a young daughter, and it really affected the stability of our life together. My world seemed much less pleasurable, and my relationships were suffering.

Thankfully, through a fortunate set of circumstances, I was led to a few people who helped me understand the nature of my symptoms. The very first thing they had me to do was cut out the refined sugars in my diet. The effects were immediate, and my health improved steadily throughout the next few months.

It was then that I began studying how diet affected my overall health and discovered one of the most important concepts I have ever learned when it comes to health. And if you get only this one thing out of this whole book, you have gotten something worthwhile. Are you ready for it? Are you sure? OK. Here it is . . .

What you eat affects your body.

Whew! There it is. I can't believe it's out there. It is like a load off of my chest. I can truly live now! I don't have to live in a closet anymore! I am free! . . . OK, so it is not *that* big of a statement. In fact, it is completely obvious. If I went around and asked people if they believed that what they ate affected their body, people would snap back with "Of course, are you an idiot?"

It's true. Think about it. We don't go around picking up rocks or chewed-up pieces of gum and popping them in our mouths to eat. We don't go to the store, buy plastic bags, rip open the box, and start chewing on the clear little baggies. That is gross! We also don't tell our kids, "Here, just eat candy bars your whole life. You seem to love them, and I want you to be happy. So from now on, the new family decree is 'chocolate bars for every meal!'"

No, we don't do this because we all know there are certain amounts of nutrients that our bodies need to receive from the food that we put in our mouths; phytonutrients that come from plants and fruits, as well as nutrients found in meats and beans.

If you need some examples of the way food affects our bodies, just look at vitamin C and how a deficiency of this vitamin causes scurvy. A few hundred years ago, scurvy was a major cause of death for those who did not have access to fruits and vegetables, especially sailors. It was an enormous problem as ships would lose up to half of their crew during a long voyage. It wasn't until a Scottish surgeon named James Lind in the British Royal Navy wrote about his experiments with scurvy that a breakthrough occurred. Lind had narrowed the cause of the disease in sailors down to a lack of citrus fruits in their diets, though we know today it to be specifically vitamin C. It took a few decades for the British navy to implement his ideas, but once they understood its effects, they began sending crates of limes on every voyage. That is where the nickname for British sailors "limey" came from. It is also one of the reasons the British navy became the most powerful sea force in the world at that time.

Another interesting example of how food affects our bodies is concerning a disease that most of us have never heard of: pellagra. In the early 1900's, pellagra was a pandemic disease that existed mostly in the southern portions of the United States. It consisted primarily of a series of symptoms that included headaches, dizziness, depression, rashes, lesions, and even insanity; all of which fell under the "umbrella" diagnosis of pellagra.

Nobody really knew the cause of pellagra until 1914, when Dr. Joseph Goldberger, a physician and epidemiologist (someone who studies epidemics), was asked to investigate this disease. Goldberg held the belief that pellagra, thought to be an infectious disease by the medical pundits of the day, was actually more of a dietary issue. After numerous, restricted-diet studies which took him many years to conduct, he was able to prove that people who consumed mostly corn-based foods and who excluded all other types of foods were at a much greater risk of having the symptoms of pellagra show up. This made logical sense, for in the South, there were many more people at that time who were living in poverty, relying solely on the corn that they grew for food.

As a cure, Dr. Goldberg urged these people to eat diets that included more of what he called "animal products" such as meat, eggs, and milk (proteins and fats). In his test studies, when the sufferers of pellagra were given diets that had these animal products, 100% of the patients recovered!

**

So the knowledge is there: *what you eat affects your body*. It's true, and it is well known. But why then do we eat things that we know are not good for us? And why do we do it every day and in such large quantities?

There are many things that we are putting into our mouths today that we shouldn't, or at least not in such great quantities — things such as processed foods, alcohol, salt, fried foods, microwaved foods, unfiltered water, pharmaceuticals, etc. But as I stated above in my list of objectives, among the purposes of this book is to focus on one particular item, refined sugar, that blessed white powder that tastes so good it makes your mouth water just thinking about it. So why am I choosing to focus on sugar? Because I believe it is one of the top uncontrolled, *legal* drugs today, and yes, I said drugs. I believe we have created a nation of sugar junkies who would rather get their daily fix than live a free, healthy life.

**

There are many physicians who tell us to limit our sugar intake, and that is what I was told by the many doctors that I visited initially. But my health never improved. It wasn't until I cut out refined sugars altogether that I saw results.

And in my search for sugar-free recipes and further information on how refined sugar affected the body, it became very apparent that there was a serious lack of resources. Most of the cookbooks that I found labeled "healthy cookbooks" focused on removing the fat and gluten but kept the refined sugars. Most of the time, I had to experiment with ingredients, taking a little from one recipe and a little from another, to come up with new recipes that did not use sugar.

In looking for further reading materials, most medical or health-related books only spoke of sugar in respect to dealing with hypoglycemia and diabetes, only recommending cutting back on sugar. Nothing I read spoke of how bad sugar was to the body and never mentioned cutting out refined sugars altogether. It was almost as if the medical community was afraid to go that far, almost as if they knew the backlash from patients would be too much. I don't blame them if that was the case.

But no matter what the reason, I imagined that if I was having these health problems, so were many others. The way I saw it, there was a hole that needed to be filled — people that needed to be helped. That was when I decided to write this book. Originally, it was intended to be just a short pamphlet for my own use when dealing with school teachers and family members who didn't understand my views on sugar. However, the more I wrote, the more I gradually became aware of how important this topic really was and how useful a book such as this would be to the countless many who are needlessly suffering from complications due to their sugar intake and addiction.

So I decided to go all out. I worked on developing what I had already put together for myself into a more succinct and practical book, complete with *The Dare*, to help those who want to take that first step.

**

Refined sugar is not just something to lessen in your life; it is something that you should eradicate from your life. It is not good at all for anyone, even in smaller amounts. My life has been greatly improved because of the information in this book. I am glad that I can share it with you, and I hope that you can help spread the word through your own success story in how you took *The Dare* and broke free from sugar addiction!

A family history of diabetes is the factor in my life which prompted me to change my habits . . . I cannot begin to tell you all the differences that I have noticed since eradicating sugar from my daily drink intake. I began by quitting sugar drinks and replacing that addiction with water. The initial result was I had a craving to compensate for the sugar I was missing. Just think, I went from 180 grams of sugar a day from drinks to "ZERO," approximately 90% of my daily sugar intake. I noticed after a few weeks, I began having more energy; my food began to taste different (better) as I lost the craving. I was able to wake up easier and earlier, but most of all, I lost forty pounds due to the change in my diet and exercise. In my opinion, sugar is a silent addiction, and everyone needs to do the research. The most important message from the diet change that I can offer is . . . "What's good to you may not be good for you."

David
Stone Mountain, GA

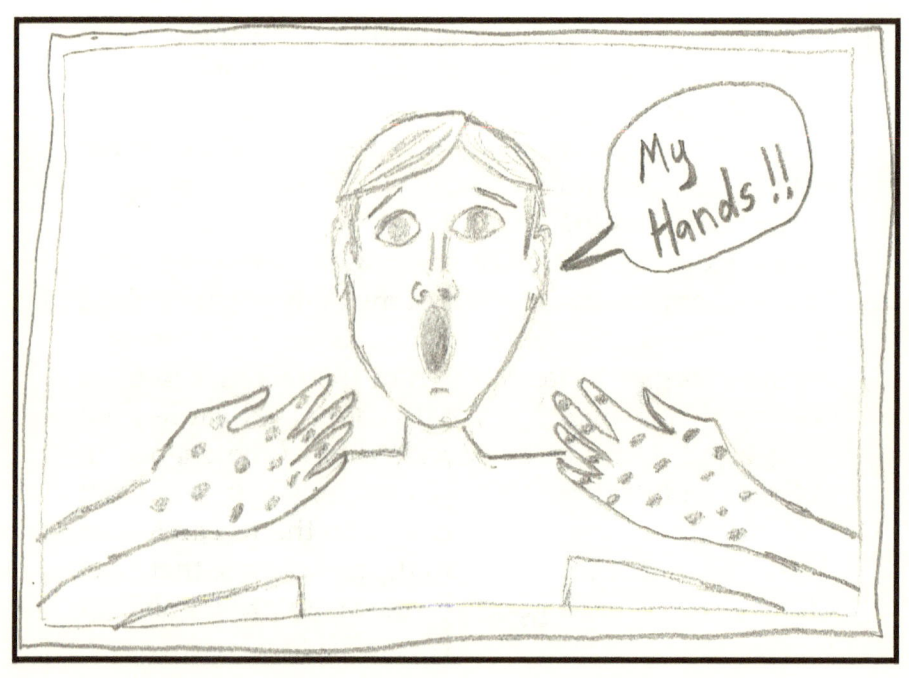

Illustration 2: This was my face upon seeing my hands.

Chapter 2: My Story

"When we are no longer able to change a situation, we are challenged to change ourselves."

—Victor Frankl

Help! I'm a mutant! What in the world? My hands were so swollen and red, I thought maybe they were going to fall off. What is going on? Am I sick, did I contract some crazy disease? Am I going to lose my hands? Maybe I touched something contagious or highly caustic, like poison ivy or some chemical. I couldn't figure it out—and I was getting really embarrassed.

You see, at the time I was working as a teacher at a local middle school. One of my duties was to supervise the In School Suspension (ISS) room for a portion of my day. ISS: that is code for, *I* can't *S*tand *S*chool. It was not a happy bunch of kids. In any case, I was sitting in the silent room one day, the kids busily pretending to work hard on their homework, all the while daydreaming about being at the beach. I was doing some grading and putting the grades into the computer when my hands started to itch. I thought nothing of it at first, just thinking it was probably some bug bites I got while being outside. But then, it kept getting worse. On top of that, my hands started to turn red and swell.

After about an hour, my hands were getting itchy. It was starting to get embarrassing as my hands didn't look normal anymore. I began to get a little worried. But it wasn't until the welts started to form all over my hands, knees, and feet that I began to panic. When I noticed this, I knew this was not just a simple bug bite or allergy. I hastily found someone to watch the kids while I went to the nurse's office. It didn't help my nerves any when the nurse took a look at my hands and gasped, "Oh my!" She then went through all the scenarios I had already gone through in my own head back in the ISS room. She said, "Maybe you touched something caustic . . . have you been around anyone with a disease lately?" We went around in circles but could not come up with a logical explanation. So she gave me some ibuprofen to try to help with the swelling and sent me on my way. I went home and immediately made a doctor's appointment for the next day.

At the doctor's office, the nurse and doctor asked all the same questions that the school nurse did; not much help there. They said that it looked like an allergic reaction and prescribed a generic antibiotic saying, "Here, let's give this a try. If it doesn't work, you can come back, pay another co-pay, and I'll give it another guess." OK, that's not exactly what they said; but that is what it felt like. I wanted a solution, not a guess.

Before I filled my prescription, I called one of my chiropractor friends and told him about my dilemma. Thank goodness I did! Most of the information that you will find in this book has stemmed from that conversation.

When I called my friend, he asked me a question that caught me off guard. He asked me what my diet was like. At the time, I didn't yet have the mindset that what I ate directly affected how I felt. So being a little impatient with my swollen hands I said, "My diet? I'm not on a diet! What does that have to do with anything?"

"No, I mean what kind of foods do you eat on a regular basis?" he replied.

"Oh," I said, "well, for starters, I get up in the morning and eat a glazed cinnamon-sugar tart; toasted. (You have to toast it to get that mm-mm good flavor — nice and warm right out of the toaster!) I usually drink that with a glass of orange juice; you know, healthy for you and full of vitamin C. Gotta keep up that immune system! Around lunch, I might grab a bite to eat at a fast food restaurant or bring a peanut butter and jelly sandwich on white bread. For dinner, it can range from a steak with mashed potatoes to a frozen dinner to Chinese food to ordering pizza."

"Well," he said, "I can't give you a professional diagnosis, but based on your current diet and from what you are describing to me about your symptoms, you might have a candida problem. One thing is for sure, your diet sure would support it."

"I could have a what problem?" I said.

"A candida problem," my friend patiently informed me. "Candida is an overgrowth of yeast in your digestive system that can cause all kinds of weird things to happen in your body, including hives, anxiety, rashes, and such."

I said, "That sounds strange. Are you sure?"

He said, "Check it out yourself. Many doctors don't believe there is such a thing as candida, but there are others who have known about it for years." Then he said something that shook the foundations of my dietary life, mainly because I didn't want to hear it . . . "And there is one thing that really feeds candida: sugar. You'll need to cut out all refined sugars for a while."

"Well, that stinks!" I thought. "Now I *am* going to have to go on a diet!"

Chances are that some of you reading this have been told by your doctor that you are diabetic and need to decrease or cut out the sugars and adopt what is commonly called a low—glycemic diet. Many of you have young children who are struggling with hyperactivity or allergies and have been told to cut out the sugars and/or gluten. Some of you would just like to lose weight and have been hearing the word about cutting carbs and simple sugars. Well, my friend telling me to cut out sugar was like telling me to stop breathing. It was what I loved!

But I valued my friend's advice and I wanted to feel better, so I got off the phone and started to do a little research on candida and diets that helped treat it. Most of my "research" was done via the Internet. And as many of you know, with all of the cure-all product advertisements and ancient healing recipes, trying to search for quality, reasonable health information is like finding a needle in a hay stack. The information was there, but it was just hard to separate the truths from the lies as well as to bring it into layman's terms.

Of course, there seemed to be a lot of scientific research done on it . . . articles written from academic and scientific studies using test groups and such. It definitely appeared to me that there was something legitimate to what my friend was telling me, at least enough for that many people to be writing about it.

So I began to attempt to change my diet. In the beginning, it was a partial change, buying what was called "wheat" bread at the store and cutting down on the candy, cakes, and pastries (when I had the will power, which was not that often). But it didn't help; I was still having the same problems. In fact, I was getting worse. I was really starting to feel bad. It wasn't just one thing like a pain in the wrist, or a cut; I was just not right and I could tell it. I started to think that I might have some sort of disease or something. I was having nausea in the mornings, throwing up a time or two just before heading off to work. I had migraine headaches. Though I'm already a thin person, I lost a little weight and began to look gaunt. I also felt a "great fatigue" coming over me; a feeling of just getting old and weak, and just slowing down. I also had a great depression come on that I couldn't shake. I couldn't handle things very well and became easily distressed.

Out of desperation, I went to see a more holistic doctor who used more natural means and who also believed that most of the ailments today are caused by poor diets and lack of exercise. I went to him and his partner nutritionist and had great success! They put me on a strict "no sugar" diet and about three or four herbal and vitamin supplements. It took me a little while to accept the diet, and I didn't do it peacefully; but once I accepted it and was faithful to the diet and to taking the herbs, the itching and swelling began to go down immediately. I actually began to have more energy and started to become a more relaxed person. On top of that, my migraine headaches that I'd been having went away. It worked! I was amazed that I started feeling the results so quickly.

Now, for those of you who have never had one before, I had what I would call a wellness experience: an experience where a health issue was cured or made much more tolerable rather than just masking the problem by a health product or a change in lifestyle. Oftentimes, these health issues are the ones that you really didn't realize you had because you've had them for so long and you just accepted them as part of your lot in life. In fact, these issues tend to define us as part of who we are—for example, we might say, "*my* allergies are flaring up" or "*my* cholesterol is high" or "*my* reflux is acting up." It is as if the symptoms are a part of you like an arm of a liver. A wellness experience usually comes after one of these health challenges gets too annoying or painful to just grit your teeth and bear it. It comes when a person seeks a solution and finds it in a manner that betters their total health.

Whether you have had a previous wellness experience or not, my hope in this book is to give everyone the chance to have their own wellness experience from the elimination of refined sugars from their diet. That is why I have put together a challenge for you, *The Dare.*

There is one more thing to add: in my particular situation, cutting out sugar wasn't the only thing I did to feel better. Depending on what ails you, in order to have a healthier life, there are other things to consider besides just sugar. Your health depends on a number of factors such as other things in your diet, genetics, good medical care, and the amount of exercise, sleep, and/or stress in your life. And though I will be discussing the one particular topic of sugar, the point I want to make from my story is that I found solutions, not temporary fixes to my health struggles. I was forcibly and reluctantly pushed out of the nest into a world more unchartered, questionable, and uncomfortable, but one with answers waiting to be uncovered. And though I appreciate doctors and highly respect their wealth of knowledge and experience, I didn't just accept their opinions as the full truth. I didn't just take the "magic pill" that was prescribed, hoping that it would make the issue just go away. This was *my* health that we were talking about.

I decided to listen to my body and learn how to help it work well on its own. This included listening to my doctor's advice, but there were other sources of information as well—books, alternative health doctors, etc. I didn't just want to medicate and treat symptoms, I wanted to be healed. I am not against pharmaceutical drugs in the right place and for the right reasons, but in my case I figured out that I wasn't having problems due to a lack of drugs in my system; so I had no reason to think that putting the drugs in my system would cure anything. If my body ever worked without problems, then it seemed to me that something happened to cause the problems; and I wanted to find out what that was. Drugs to me were like spraying water on the flames of a fire instead of at the base; it looks like you are doing something, but the water is just evaporating and the flames grow bigger and bigger. Treating symptoms just allows the source of the problems to grow larger.

In my case, I discovered that I am genetically predisposed to such things as hypoglycemia, diabetes, and even depression and psychosis. That is the part that I cannot change. I can't ask God to give me a different body. But I did discover that I could change my lifestyle. Had I continued in the path I was going, I probably would have deteriorated more and more into an unhealthy state, developing more issues that increased with time. I fully believe that I'd be a diabetic by now, knowing my family history and how my body reacts to sugars. But I didn't continue that path. I didn't just give in to my doctor's advice to medicate and hope for the best. I actively sought answers that worked. I went on a journey to find those answers that would make me feel better permanently.

I'm not promising that if you already have cancer or suffer from heart disease, that you can be healed by cutting out sugar.* Disease

_____

*   If you would like a more comprehensive guide to maximize your health, there is a great book called *The Optimal Health Revolution* by Dr. Duke Johnson. It gives a wonderful overview of what Dr. Johnson calls the "Eight Pillars of Optimal Health." Dr. Johnson has discovered some amazing connections between our lifestyles

often comes from years of abusive habits. And cutting out sugar one week won't cure all disease. However, I sincerely believe that cutting refined sugar out of your diet will make you feel better, think better, and live better. I would love to see many of the sad, hopeless faces out there regain the hope that is available through good health because much of the time your health directs your moods which affects your entire life.

(mainly diet) and the most common chronic diseases of today and the underlying factor, inflammation.

I was diagnosed with diabetes four years ago by (the hospital on) the weekend. On the Monday prior to my diagnosis, I fainted while on my feet . . . on two separate occasions. In addition, I experienced extreme dehydration and blurred vision; the blurred vision was noticeable starting on the Wednesday before.

At the hospital, the doctors told me that I was very lucky to make it into the ER when I did because, if I would have passed out, I probably would have died from a sugar-induced coma. My sugar level was 995 when my glucose was checked by the triage nurse.

After a five-day stay at the facility I was told that I would have to take the insulin the rest of my life. I was taught to give myself a shot three times a day every day before every meal and given a glucose test kit to check my sugar levels after every meal. A number for the nutritionist was provided and it was suggested that I attend a class. Making that phone call and talking with others who recently shared similar experiences proved fruitful in a matter of speaking.

I learned to understand how to read food labels which led to a change on my outlook of food. Food is no longer a sport for me. I no longer eat because a certain food group looks and smells good. I now treat food more like toothpaste, a means to an end. I only need to eat to satisfy my body's needs and ignore or dismiss everything I was taught or learned before about food and eating.

My diet change included the following:

- No white flour
- No processed sugar foods or snacks — snacks are fruits and (whole wheat) crackers only.
- No soda of any kind — water and diet tea only.

Continued on next page . . .

- I eat three meals a day with snacks in-between. Breakfast, to this day, is still two packets of oatmeal and a cup of peach/mango tea. Lunch and dinner are home-cooked and include meat, veggies, and a starch of small to medium portion.
- In the beginning, if I was not full from the meal, I would follow up with fruit of any kind and more water to feel full.

The above changes were implemented about six months after the original diagnosis. After changing my diet, I was able to switch from the liquid insulin that was administered by me three times a day to the pill form . . .

After one year of taking pills to regulate my sugar levels I started to notice that my sugar was regulating before I could take my medication. For example, I would know my sugar is getting low because I would start to feel a little shaky and agitated before it was time to eat again.

I stopped taking the insulin on my own, not recommended, but I trusted the message my body was sending to me. I felt that my body was telling me to leave the processed food alone and that I would be OK. I did just that; and two months ago my doctor told me that I can live a normal life without medication as long as I'm responsible with eating habits.

Please understand that although diabetes has some history in my family, mine was habit-induced. I honestly feel that my body changed once I changed my habits. My dad passed away in December of 2011 of cancer; he was diagnosed a diabetic fifteen years before he passed away. He too was able to control his diabetes through eating habits and had not taken insulin for the last eight years of his life.

Ron
Duluth, GA, by way of Jamaica Queens

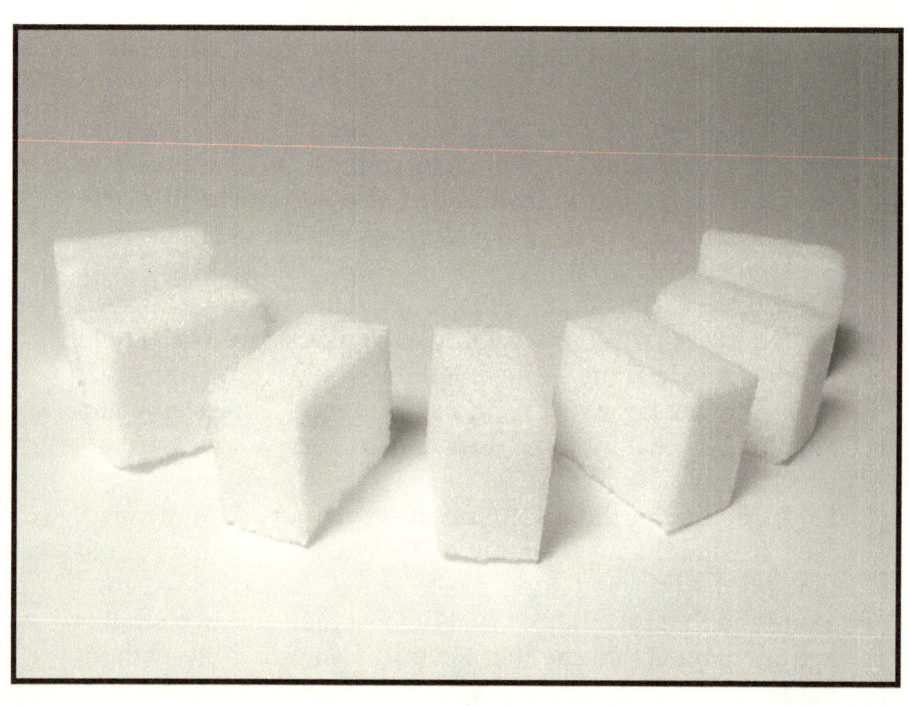

Illustration 3: lumps of table sugar (sucrose).

Chapter 3: Sugar 101: Homeostasis

"¹SUG·AR \ 'shŭge(r)\ n—**1a.** *a sweet, crystallizable substance that consists entirely or essentially of sucrose, that is colorless or white when pure and usually yellowish to brown otherwise, that occurs naturally in the most readily available amounts in sugarcane, sugar beets, sugar maple, sorghum, and sugar palms, that is obtained commercially principally by processing the juice expressed from sugarcane or the aqueous extract of sliced sugar beets and refined* so that the final product is the same regardless of the source, and that forms an important article of human food and is used also chiefly as a condiment and preservative for other foods and for drugs and in the chemical industry as an intermediate.* **1b** . . . . ᵗ"*

So what is sugar? Well, for the purpose of our discussion, I am going to place sugar into two categories. The first is *unrefined* sugar. This is the natural, God-created substance that is found in whole foods such as apples, grapes, carrots, tomatoes, and beets. We are supposed to eat these foods. Our bodies can produce many things used for regular function. But there are many other things such as vitamins, minerals, *and sugars* that our bodies do not produce and which we need to eat to get. These natural foods come from the earth. Genesis 1:29 says, "Behold I have given you every plant yielding seed that is on the face of the earth, and every tree with seed in its fruit. You shall have them for food." So we are supposed to eat them.

The type of sugar in fruits is called fructose. In many plants, it is glucose or sucrose (the type that comes from the sugar beet or sugarcane). Glucose is also what the carbohydrates (including table sugar) we eat turn into and passes throughout our bodies to fuel our cells. The sugar in dairy is called lactose.

In general, these sugars are not at all bad to eat as you are getting plenty of fiber and nutrients along with the sugar. Also, you are

---

ᵗ   Webster's Third International Dictionary of the English Language, Unabridged — 1993. Italics were added for emphasis.

not getting massive doses of the sugar at one time when you are eating a plant or a piece of fruit. Sugar is necessary for the human body to function. Unrefined sugars coming from the foods we eat are a great source of energy and they taste very sweet to those unaccustomed to the other category of sugar.

The other category on which I am placing the term "sugar" is *refined sugar*. This is the "sweet, crystallized substance" mentioned in the definition above as "able to be turned into dry crystals that can be put into little packets for use." This type of sugar comes out of a purification or refining process. This process removes everything but the sweet liquid portion of the plant and then processes and purifies this liquid.

The type of refined sugar mostly consumed is in the form of table sugar (sucrose), usually coming from sugarcane or sugar beets but in a much more concentrated form than the plant. Another common type of refined sugar widely used is a combination of fructose and glucose (otherwise known as corn syrup).[‡] Please pardon the pun, but of the two categories of sugar, refined sugar is the type that Americans are just "eating up!" In fact, according to a 1999 Center for Science in the Public Interest poll, the average per-person consumption of added, refined sugar has gone up 28% since 1986 from 127 pounds per year to 155.6 pounds per year by 1998.[§] I'm curious to know if that includes all of the sugar used in processed foods as a preservative! Another statistic states that at the turn of the century in 1900, the average person ate only ninety pounds a year. It also says that in 1800, it was eighteen pounds a year and only four pounds a year in 1700.[¶]

[‡] ˙As a side note, though it comes from natural sources, I would place honey as a refined sugar based on what it does once in the body. In terms of its make-up, honey is a solution of about 80% glucose, fructose, and sucrose with 20% water.

[§] http://www.cspinet.org/reports/sugar/sugarpet1.pdf

[¶] Article from www.Mercola.com: http://articles.mercola.com/sites/articles/archive/2010/04/20/sugar-dangers.aspx

Just to put these numbers into perspective, one hundred and fifty-eight pounds a year is just under one-half a pound a day, which is slightly under one cup, or sixteen tablespoons. Most sodas have around three and one-third tablespoons of sugar in a twelve-ounce can; so you are looking at about five sodas worth of sugar a day, every day! That is what the average American is putting in their bodies.

So from now on in this book, when you hear me mention the term "sugar," I am not referring to unrefined, natural sugar found in whole, unprocessed foods. I am referring to refined sugar. This is the form of sugar that is harming us as individuals and as a society, and it is the only type of sugar that we will be discussing in this book.

**

Whether you know much about cars or not, I think most people would understand if I said the body is like a shiny new car with numerous working parts that constantly need maintenance and fuel. With the car, we take it for an oil change or have the tires rotated to maintain its integrity and longevity. For the body, the maintenance might be such things as exercise, rest, and perhaps some time at the doctor's for checkups or medication to help healing.

In terms of the fuel, our body only needs three things for it to function: *oxygen, water,* and *food*. One of these things, we get by breathing. The other two we get by ingesting: eating and drinking. I'm pretty sure that most people don't have any problems knowing how to breathe or remembering to do so. But many of us do have trouble remembering the importance of what we put into our mouths. What goes in our mouths is, among other things, our fuel that moves the machine. And like all machines it can either be running optimally (as good as it can), or it can be running somewhere less than optimal. This is basic stuff, I know, but bear with me.

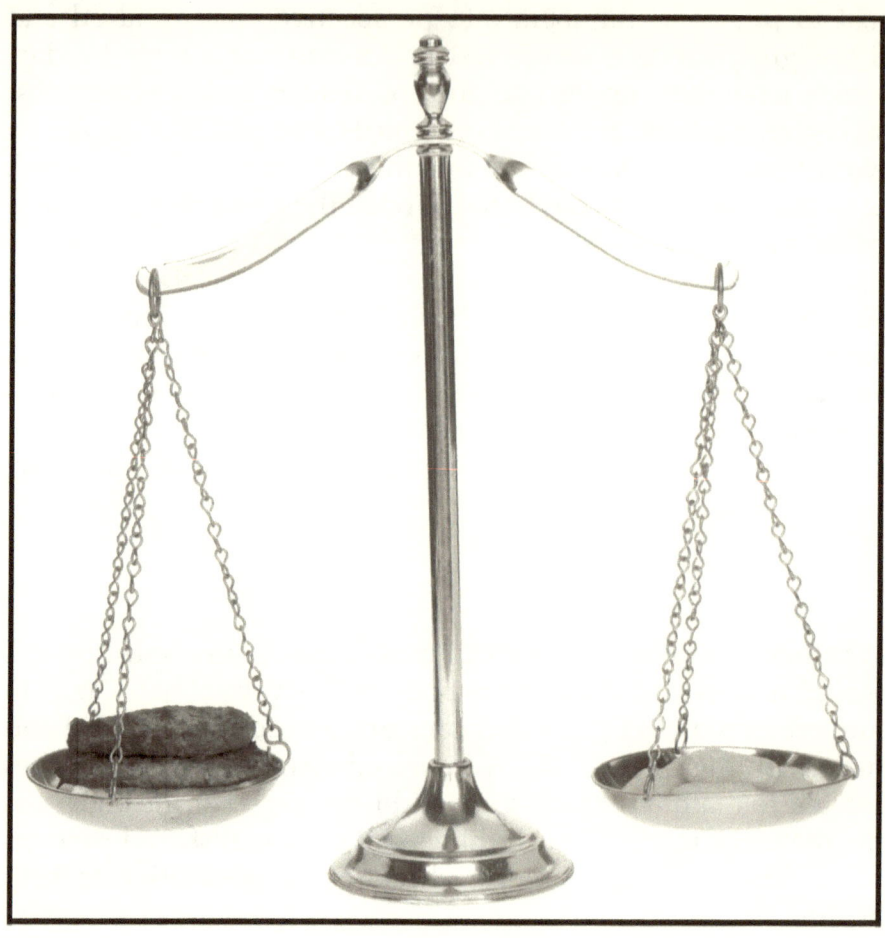

Illustration 4: a balance scale.

**

When I was in school I learned a great word in anatomy and physiology, *homeostasis (hoe-mee-o-stae-sis)*, which means having a balance in the body. I like this word. It means that for the body to function it can never have too much of any one thing, or too little. It is amazing that the body is so intricate, with so many chemicals and electrical functions that all work simultaneously. In fact, the body is so amazing that in just a small paper cut, there are around forty chemicals that have to enter the bloodstream and reach that paper cut in just the right amounts, in just the right order, and at just the right time to keep us from bleeding to death. If any one of those chemicals is out of place or not the right amount, you have a bleeding disorder and are at risk. There are some chemicals, like serotonin, that affect the body in such a way that if there is just a slight variation, the person begins to have all kinds of problems, including insomnia, depression, loss of memory, anxiety, and a host of other issues.

Balance is the way of the world. If you think about it, balance is the way of all of God's creation — ecosystems, weather, government, etc. Balance is also important in our interpersonal relationships: marriage, work, play. Trouble comes when imbalance occurs, when you have too much of one thing and not enough of another.

This is also applicable when dealing with our machinelike bodies. When the body is running optimally, everything is *in* balance. When it is not running optimally, things are *out-of* balance. Take that shiny new car that you were thinking of earlier. Think of the problems that occur when the parts of the car are out of balance: the tires need an alignment and rotation, the engine needs a tune-up, the engine has too much buildup on the inside causing the fuel and air mixture to be off, etc. If the car is too far out of balance, you might be one of those people on the side of the road with a real nice — looking car that doesn't work.

For those of you who don't like cars, picture trying to make a cake where you don't have *all* the ingredients; but you have *most* of them. Imagine going ahead and making that cake with half the oil or replacing some of the sugar with salt. What about only using one egg instead of two? You are still making that cake, right? You can still put some icing on it to make it look good, but just wait and look at the face of the person who tries it. It would be entertaining at best. The recipe was written because *all* ingredients were balanced properly and meant to be included.

And what happens to a life that is not in balance? What if you focused so much on work that you ignored your girlfriend, spouse, or kids? What if you focus so much on pleasure and entertainment that you never take care of the things that need to get done? You start to suffer. **Homeostasis**! Balance is key; not too much of one thing and yet not too little.

So how does the body keep this homeostasis? Well, as I said, the human body is a wonderful creation that is comprised of numerous elements and which produces hundreds of chemicals and millions of electrical impulses that work together in harmony to allow a human being to be able to do such things as think, chew, walk, see, and talk. It is an amazing creation when you think of it all working together without an ounce of effort on our part! And within each of these creations, there is a balance that the body wants to keep. Though everything is not always in balance, the body is constantly seeking to maintain this equilibrium. That is how health is achieved.

Take the hormone adrenaline, for instance. The body uses adrenaline to create the necessary energy needed in emergency situations. Scientists call this the "fight or flight" response. It's what gives you that extra burst of energy you need.

You are walking down the path in the woods; you come around a big boulder only to be face to face with a very large, smelly, not-so-intelligent grizzly bear. You turn and run with a vigor that you've never had before. Why? Because if you don't, you are going to be dinner! Inside your body, when you first see the bear, the adrenal glands immediately inject adrenaline into your bloodstream. The blood moves so fast that it literally takes just a few seconds for the adrenaline to spread throughout the body and to feel the effects.

So by the time you actually see the bear, realize the danger, and turn around to run, you are feeling the adrenaline in your system. Among other things, the adrenaline speeds up your heart rate, increases your blood pressure, diverts more blood to the muscles and away from the brain, and dilates your pupils. There is not much rational thinking going on when you are in flight mode, but the body is getting more energy and oxygen to do its job because of adrenaline.

But what happens once the threat is over? Optimally, the body will eliminate the adrenaline from the blood and the person will calm down, going back into equilibrium. Again, the body is seeking this balance, which is the healthiest state to be in.

When it comes to sugars, there is a certain amount of sugar that needs to be in our blood in order for the body to have a nice, steady supply of energy. When we eat foods such as a piece of whole wheat toast or cracker (which are complex carbohydrates) the carbohydrates are broken down into sugar for the body's cells to use. The process begins in the mouth, as the person is chewing. Enzymes in the saliva start breaking down the food, since the food is in its natural form (wheat) and the sugar is bound up in with the fiber. The enzymes have to be pulled out of the usable parts of the food. Some of the nutrients are absorbed immediately, including any glucose (sugar) that has already been broken down, but the rest travels down into the stomach.

In the stomach, the acids break down the food even more. As the food passes into your small intestine a little at a time, more and more of the converted food is absorbed into the bloodstream to travel to every cell of your body. As the glucose (and other nutrients) are slowly pulled out of the food and absorbed into the blood, this small increase of glucose spreads throughout the body. As it reaches the control center of the body, the brain is informed of the increase and decides that it better make sure that this increase in glucose is controlled and does not get out of hand. So it sends a signal to the pancreas to produce a chemical called insulin, which tells the liver, muscles, and fat tissues to use up the sugar. This helps regulate the balance of the body and allow the cells to get the energy they need.

The body then uses up the glucose ("burning" it or storing it), the blood moves back to its normal levels, and everything balances back out. After some time, as the cells in the body start wanting more energy, this person starts to have that feeling of hunger we all get. This prompts the person to go to the cabinet, pull out something else to eat, and take a bite. The process starts all over again, and the cells get fed. This is how the body is supposed to work, like an engine running optimally; a well-oiled machine; a perfectly made cake. It is a brilliant system and so delicately balanced.

Homeostasis! Remember that word. It's a great word!

I was a junk food and convenience food addict for most of my life. I also *loved, loved, loved* sweets! I would bake a cake just to eat most of it by myself. I'd whip up a batch of frosting just to eat it out of the bowl! I could never just eat one or two cookies. I had to have the entire batch of them! I was out of control. As a result, I rode the waves of being up, only to crash a little while later leading to yet more sugar cravings and a repeat of the cycle. I was depressed and tired all the time. My brain felt like it was constantly filled with fog and my productivity was on a steady decline. I did not want to go on like that anymore, so I went on a quest to improve my heath through diet and eventually transitioned to a raw-foods lifestyle. I cut out all the refined sugar in my diet and what a difference that made in my life. I found that once I got over the addiction (and it *is* an addiction), I was happier, and the depression that had kept me trapped for so long started to lift. I also finally knew what it felt like to have true energy. Not the kind brought about by the intake of toxic substances but energy that radiates from inside your body all day long without the ups and downs that the artificial stuff gives you. Other amazing benefits I experienced were clear thinking and weight loss! No more foggy brain and extra jiggle around my waist. Who doesn't want that? I was able to be more productive and actually accomplish any objective I wanted. Now all my sugar comes from fruits! Delicious, juicy, filled with nutrition fruit! As a holistic health coach, one of the first things I advise my clients to do is to stop eating refined sugar. While sometimes it may be a struggle because refined sugar is in almost all of our packaged products, they are always amazed at how much better they (and their families) feel afterwards. My recommendation is the next time you need a sugar fix, reach for an apple!

Shannon Kilbourn
Atlanta, GA
Holistic Health Coach
www.takechargewellness.com

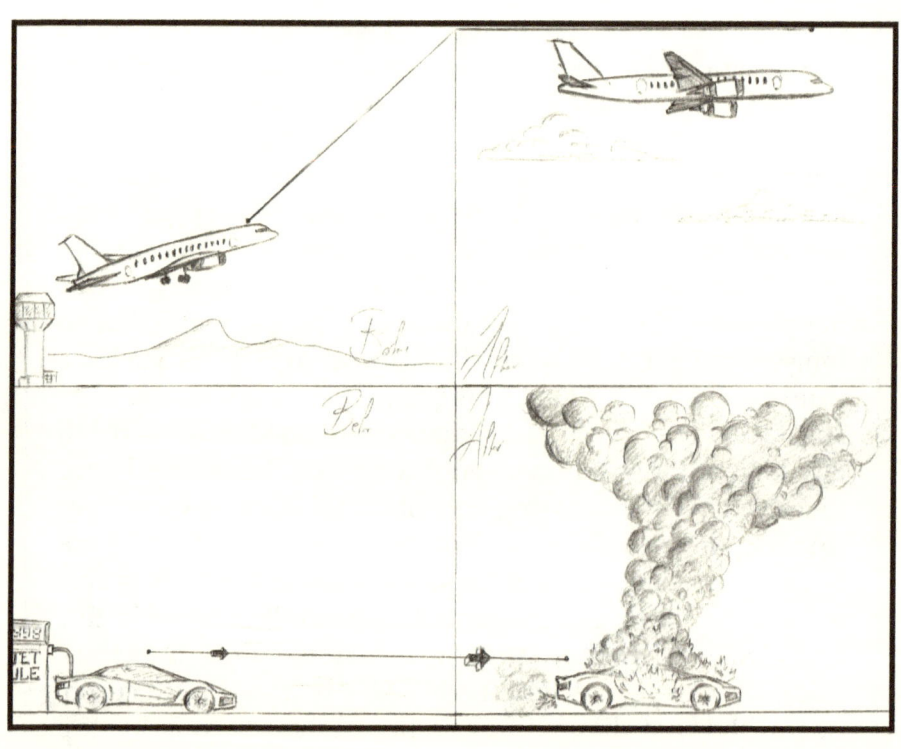

Illustration 5: Cars are not meant to use jet fuel and vice versa. Man is not meant for refined sugars.

Chapter 4: Burnout, Deficiency, and Inflammation

Journal of the American Medical Association (JAMA)

"In combination, in (the year) 2000 dietary patterns and sedentary lifestyles represent the most common source of unnecessary death and disease among Americans, with a range from 340,000 to 642,000 deaths annually."

Source: *http://www.rwjf.org/reports/grr/032016.htm*
Robert Wood Johnson Foundation
"Poor Diets, Little Exercise Leading Cause of Preventable Illness and Deaths"

In chapter three, we discussed the normal process of how the body maintains homeostasis and health. Now, let's talk about what happens to the body when a person eats refined sugar and disrupts this balance. When I discovered what sugar physically did to my body, I immediately wanted to cut it out of my diet. However, I found it to be a lot harder than I thought. It was both my physical and psychological addictions to sugar that made it hard. We will discuss the addictiveness of sugar a little later.

When I thought about writing this book, I didn't want to proclaim a problem without providing a solution. I also didn't want to throw out a quickly-put-together gimmicky solution that nobody would follow or that didn't produce results. My plan with this book is to make it much easier on you who want to take *The Dare* and make the change. I want to empower you with all of the information and tools you need to be successful.

For me, I decided to take *The Dare* because my body was physically breaking down. I was having real problems that were interfering with my day-to-day life. Many of you might not have such problems, and I hope you don't. But I also hope that by providing you with my story and more specific information on what is happening inside your body when you eat refined sugars, you will get a glimpse of what can and probably will, at some point, happen if you continue to consume large amounts of refined, processed sugars. A very successful man I know once said, "It is kind of like going out to a landing strip and standing to one side of the runway then walking in a straight line across to the other side of the runway, doing a 180-degree turnaround, and walking straight back to where you started." My friend says, "If you will do this over and over, and if you will do this long enough, there is one thing that I can almost guarantee you will happen . . . you're going to get hit by an airplane." Many of us are walking across the flight line when it comes to our health, and sooner or later, the plane is going to come by in the form of illness.

I don't think it is just a sheer coincidence that our population's obesity rates are skyrocketing or that the numbers of chronic diseases like diabetes, arthritis, and asthma are at all-time highs at the same time that our lives are becoming more sedentary and our diets more full of processed foods and sugars. What amazes me is how so little attention is paid to the average person's daily diet and how these poor diets are affecting our health individually and as a nation. And if a nation is not healthy, it creates many more problems.

The following description is a very simplified version of how the body works. If you are a scientist, forgive my lack of scientific terminologies and exact details. The point is not to explain all functions involved but to gain a general understanding of what is going on inside. I want to show the reason why taking *The Dare* is important and how it just might save you from getting hit by that 747.

**

Picture yourself dressed in the clown outfit, red nose and large floppy shoes. You're out with your children on the one night of the year that most parents give the free-for-all "go-ahead" on the candy consumption—Halloween. We reason, "I did it when I was a kid . . . so why not?" I love what Jerry Seinfeld says about kid's reactions to this event. Here's a little snippet from *I'm Telling You for the Last Time*:

> "Candy was my whole life when I was a kid. The first ten years of my life, I think the only clear thought I had was 'GET CANDY!' That was it. Family, friends, school—they are just obstacles in the way of candy. I'm out for the candy here. I'm just thinking 'get candy, get candy, get candy . . .'" That's why you have to teach kids not to take candy from a stranger when they are playing on a playground; because they are such (crazy brained) that they are like (in a robotic voice) 'this man has candy. Goodbye, I don't care what happens to me. Get candy, get candy, get candy.'" . . . So the first time you hear the concept of Halloween, your brain can't even process the information. You're like (in a shocked voice), "What is this? What did you say? What did you say about giving out candy? Who's giving out candy? Everyone that we *know* is just giving out candy! Are you kidding me? When is this happening? Where? Take me with you! I've got to be a part of this! I'll do anything that they want! . . . I can wear that."**

That is so true! I remember loving trick-or-treating when I was a kid and eating so much candy that I thought I was going to die. Today, we are the parents taking out our own children. We take them throughout the neighborhood, going door to door until we have bags that are bursting with candy. Then we take this "booty" that we've collected and pour it out on the table at home. We grab one of our kid's pieces of candy under the guise of a safety check and put it in our mouth. We call it a taste test. Besides the extreme pleasure that we get in our mouth, here is what is happening inside our body . . .

** Jerry Seinfeld, *I'm Telling You for the Last Time*

Being that this is not a piece of fruit with fiber or a piece of whole grain bread that will slowly be digested, this piece of candy is dissolved in my mouth and stomach and quickly absorbed in the intestines within twenty minutes. Being that it is sucrose, which is very similar to glucose, it mostly skips the process of digestion. My blood does not get a steady flow of sugar but rather a big shot of it. As my body does its normal job of regulating the blood sugar levels it starts creating the insulin to tell the cells to burn the sugar. But there is something very wrong here. This is not a normal amount of sugar in the blood; this is a very large amount.

Now my body is in a state of emergency! My pancreas immediately goes into overdrive and pumps out large amounts of insulin to speedily process the sugars. It works, and the blood sugar levels begin to go down. (Meanwhile, I'm enjoying the "sugar high.") And because there is much more glucose available than the body can possibly use for energy, the liver turns the extra into fat. It's no wonder I find myself continually gaining a little extra weight every year!

As this mini-party that is going on inside my body begins to calm down, I begin to experience what is commonly called "a sugar crash." The insulin did its job well and is getting rid of all the excess sugar in my blood. The problem is that now, there was so much insulin created that my sugar level drops to a level below homeostasis, sometimes dangerously low. I start to get sluggish, easily irritated, or plain grumpy.

For a person like me, the reaction might be more extreme, as I am a person who genetically struggles with metabolizing sugars. But in eating the piece of candy, I begin to feel the effects and am starting to feel hungry even though I just gave myself a lot of calories. My body tells me that I need to eat to replace the missing blood sugar and get back homeostasis. My body senses this as an emergency, since a lack of sugar in my system literally starves my tissues and organs and prevents them from working properly.

So in this state of frenzied hunger, what do you think we all do at this point? — We eat something, typically something that either

has added sugar for taste or has been preserved with sugar. This
starts the whole process over again.

Here is the major problem with this scenario. It is not that our
bodies are not doing their job. Yes, the body is working when
it filters out this poison that we are putting in our bodies. The
problem is how many times we make our bodies do this. The
average American puts their body through this cycle at least three
times a day, seven days a week, fifty-two weeks a year! In reality,
I would guess the number is more likely up to ten times a day,
considering how much candy we eat, the sugar in our coffee, the
doughnuts at work, the sugary snacks from the vending machine
throughout the day, and the pie for a late-night snack. And it is
having a negative effect on our health.

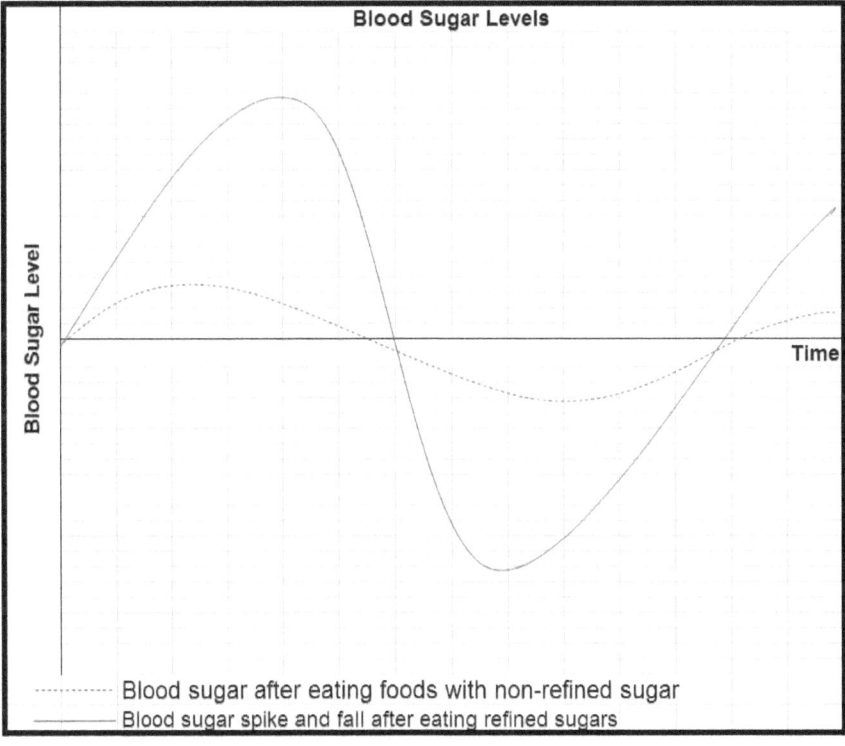

Illustration 6: This is a graph of blood sugar levels over time. You can see
that the blood sugar swings a lot more up and down when we eat refined
sugars. It is no wonder our pancreas gives out on us!

**

The Dare is about eliminating refined sugar from your diet for a temporary period of time — one month. But I am not saying that eating refined sugar every once in a while (once you are done with taking *The Dare* of course!) will kill a person. It is not that a person can't ever eat refined sugar. If I'm out with a group, every once in a while, I might eat a piece of cheesecake with sugar in it, and I haven't died yet. But there is great book called *The Compound Effect*, by the publisher of *Success Magazine* Darren Hardy, which says that success and failure are not found in one great event but in the compounded effects of hundreds or thousands of small, seemingly insignificant decisions or habits.[††]

My first taste of this was when I was in elementary school. My school had a man come in to talk to us about smoking. I say "talk," though this person really couldn't talk because he had no larynx. It was taken out due to throat cancer which the doctors believed was directly caused by his smoking habit. He usually kept a covering around his neck; but for our education, he took it off to show us a gaping hole in his throat. He was able to use something that looked like a kazoo that he would hold up to the hole and "speak" with; but because of the fact that he had no vocal chords, he had no ability to vary his pitch. He sounded like a Martian saying, "Take me to your leader." It was very impactful to me as a child, and I remember everything that he said. He told us that it all started with the first cigarette. Needless to say, that very day I decided that smoking was not a habit I wanted to take up. Even when I experimented with smoking in high school, I always had that picture in my mind of the hole in that man's neck. Eating one doughnut or cookie is not going to make you a diabetic, give you high blood pressure, or osteoporosis just like smoking one cigarette will not give you throat cancer. However, a regular habit of eating doughnuts and cookies with refined sugars will eventually cause problems. It is the cumulative effect of this habit that damages the body over time. And that is exactly what

---

[††]   *The Compound Effect*, Darren Hardy. SUCCESS Media. 2010.

is happening to us as a nation. We as Americans have created a habit of eating sugar in almost everything we eat.

If I were to discuss in depth the full effects of this habit on our bodies, I would end up with a book the size of a college textbook. I highly doubt most people would read it and frankly, it is not necessary. We don't all need to know how the car works to use it. Just a few basic concepts like how to use the key and how to change the gears are enough. When it comes to how a diet that is high in sugar affects the body, I believe that we only need to discuss three core issues. Why just three? Because I believe these are the three underlying, foundational issues that all other issues stem from. It is like working on a building that has made it through a bad earthquake but is about to fall due to some major cracks in the foundation and the structure. Your job is to repair the building in order to keep it from falling. You can work on the upper floors all you want but until you make sure that the cracked and weakened foundation is fixed, the whole structure is likely to fall. These three issues that stem from eating refined sugar in our diet are the cracks in the foundation that affect the whole building that is our body. They are called **burnout, deficiency, and inflammation**.

**

BURNOUT

Drinking sodas and sweet coffees, eating sugary cereals and sweet deserts, and munching on sugary candy throughout the day is like taking your brand new car, driving to the gas station, opening up the gas tank, and then pumping jet fuel into the tank. Oh, the car runs great for a short while; but it will sustain an enormous amount of strain and wear in the process.‡‡ At first, your car will

---

‡‡ In reality, jet fuel would not have this effect. It would gum up the engine quickly without burning hot. The "burnout" I speak of would more likely come from burning alcohol or a higher octane fuel in the engine. I just used jet fuel for the imagery that people associate it with.

act like a race car with lots of power; this would be a good time to race the pimple-faced teenager in his little road-racer! But in a short while, the engine is going to start breaking down. The jet fuel burns too hot and burns up the insides of the engine, melting all seals and gaskets that are essential for the engine to work. You'll get ahead of the teenager's road-racer only to find yourself on the side of the road with a melted engine. That is what I mean by burnout, when something that was once working no longer is because the wrong substance was used, ingested, or applied.

Now if you are not a car person, you can visualize burnout a few other ways, too. When I bought my first house, I was very excited to have my own lawn. I watered it, kept it cut, and made sure that it was well fed. I guess my belief was that the more you gave your lawn food and water, the greener it would be. But I got a little overzealous with the fertilizer. The lawn looked nice for a little while, but that was right before it turned yellow and then died. I had put too much fertilizer on my lawn and burned it up.

Eating refined sugar is also like putting too much bleach in your washer. If you dilute the bleach in the washer, you can safely bleach your clothes. But if you soak your clothes in pure bleach for any amount of time, it will quickly begin to break down the clothing, and holes and other major signs of wear will begin to appear. Why? Because bleach is an acid, and it is literally burning up your clothes.

When we consistently eat or drink refined sugars, the effects resemble the burnout of our body. Just like the engine that quit, the grass that died, and the clothes that burned up, our internal organs and tissues can burn out as well. The example at the beginning of this chapter of the blood-sugar cycle and how it leads to such issues as diabetes is just one example of this. After continual blood sugar emergencies, the pancreas becomes less and less effective in maintaining the blood sugar homeostasis. In chapter five, I will discuss diabetes more in depth as well as other examples of burnout including kidney damage, a weakened immune system, and cardiovascular disease. But at this point, just remember that one of the core effects of regular sugar intake is having things stop working when they once were. That is burnout.

Much of burnout occurs because of the concentrated amounts of sugar that we eat. Have you ever eaten sour candy? If so, you are familiar with the mouth-puckering effects. Taken one at a time, each piece of candy is tolerable and fun. One of my wife's college friends found out that you can purchase the sour substance in concentrated form. Apparently, after buying the concentrated sour chemical, they had the "great" idea of putting the stuff on the mouthpieces of all their fellow band members. Of course, my wife's friend picked the most opportune time, right before a performance. Not only did it make their mouths pucker, but it was uncontrollable and could not be stopped for at least thirty minutes. Ouch! My wife never heard what happened when the band director found out, but I can only imagine that he or she wasn't too happy. Just imagine what would have happened if someone had drank the liquid!

But that is what we do every day. We are "drinking the liquid." This is why refined sugar affects our bodies the way it does, because it is in a concentrated form, just like the sour stuff, the undiluted bleach, and the jet fuel. Refined sugar is the by-product of a process that takes something that grows naturally (like the sugarcane or sugar beet) and takes everything healthy out of it, leaving a totally nutrition-less, but very tasty, substance. In all of life, if you take something that is naturally occurring and you increase the quantity and/or magnify it numerous times, it becomes dangerous. Chances are the lip-puckering substance my wife's friend was toying with was a concentrated amount of something natural and harmless in its original form. Look at citric acid, found in the common orange. Take an orange and juice it and the kids have a nice glass of OJ. Take the juice and purify it until you have concentrated citric acid and now you have the stuff that we clean the kitchen with that smells so "citrusy." It cleans well, but is not meant for consumption—neither appealing nor healthy.

How about sunlight? Sunlight is a very healthy thing, but get too much of it and you can get cancer. Focus and magnify sunlight and you get a laser, capable of burning things at a much higher temperature and in less time, like when we used to burn leaves or ants as a child

What about an apple? Apples are healthy, right? After all, an apple a day keeps the doctor away. Take that apple and put it in a press to take out all the fiber and what do you get? Apple juice. I love apple juice! Though you don't have the fiber anymore, you are still getting a lot of vitamin C. If you create a "mush" out of the apples and let it ferment and filter out the solids, what do you have? Apple wine. Purify it one more time and you get brandy. Now, some of you might like a little nightcap here and there; but unfortunately, now there is no fiber and no nutrition for you at all. In fact, if you drink enough of it, your liver will burn out as well. Well, let's go a little further; ferment it some more and what do you get . . . rubbing alcohol, or something like it. Don't try drinking rubbing alcohol. It will kill you!

It is the same with sugar. If you take the sugarcane plant or sugar beet and you chop it up or steam it, you have a good tasting vegetable that you can eat and is healthy. You have vitamins and minerals from the soil and you have fiber along with the unrefined sugar. But take that beet, purify it over and over again and you have a concentrated substance that, if ingested on a regular basis, causes health issues and even death. Go back and reread the definition of sugar. It is not only used as a food condiment, but is also used in the manufacturing of drugs and as a preservative. Have you ever wondered why sugar can be used as a preservative? If bacteria don't even like sugar, what do you think it does to our bodies? This is burnout.

**

DEFICIENCY

When I say takeout, I don't mean picking up your favorite Chinese food from the restaurant down the street. What I mean by takeout is the removal of a substance which in turn causes damage. The body has many chemicals, minerals, and vitamins that it needs to function. We either get these from the foods we eat or our bodies produce them. But when you start taking one or more of these substances away, there is a gap in the body's ability to function. This is known as a deficiency: a shortage of substances necessary to health.[§§]

When I was a kid, Steven Spielberg produced a movie called *The Dark Crystal*. At the time, it was a spectacle of modern special effects. The plot involved a character Jen, who was destined to save his people, the Gelflings, and return order and harmony to the world. In the movie, the Gelflings are enslaved to evil creatures called Skeksis. One of the things these evil creatures did was to attach these Gelflings to a machine that would suck the living "essence" out of the Gelfling. Then, the Skeksis would drink the liquid essence. This is what kept the Skeksis from aging and dying. The sad part is that it would also turn the Gelfling into a gaunt, lifeless, slave of a creature. The body would still be alive, but the eyes and cheeks would be sunk in, the skin color would go pale, and the living spirit of the Gelfling would be gone. When there is a deficiency in the body, just like the Gelfling's body, it becomes weak and lifeless because something (the essence) is not there or is being pulled out of the body — sucked out. Sugar generally has an effect just like this; it acts like the Skesis, sucking the essential substances from the body.

One of the things that a diet in refined sugars affects is the calcium in our bones. Along with weight-bearing activity, calcium is what makes bones strong. Calcium is not something that the body creates on its own. We get it through the foods we eat and then it is stored in the bones. If individuals don't get enough calcium in their diet, especially when they are young, they are more prone to breaking bones and to such issues as osteoporosis as they get older. But if calcium is being taken out of the body for some reason, the effects are even worse.

[§§] Merriam-Webster's School Dictionary, 2004. p. 248.

When a woman has a baby, she has to provide calcium to the new baby's skeleton and other functions as the baby grows in the womb. This is why many women take supplements during pregnancy. If the mother is not eating food rich in calcium or not supplementing calcium in her diet, her body will take it from her own bones, leaving her bones and teeth weak and prone to disease. This is one of the reasons that women are more prone to osteoporosis than men. Women typically begin life with lower bone density and also lose bone mass faster than men with age. They also generally reach their peak bone mass at eighteen; and by age thirty, their bones are "fully stocked" with the maximum calcium reserves that it will ever have. From then on, they are in a steady state of losing bone density.

So where does sugar come into the picture? Most people have a hard time imagining how eating sugar can affect such things as osteoporosis. But like all things in the world, everything in the body is connected. When one area is affected, it causes a chain reaction that affects other areas and eventually the whole body. There was a study done by a physician in Britain, Dr. John Yudkin, that directly connects the health of bones to sugar. Dr. Yudkin's study shows much higher levels of a chemical called cortisol in the fasting bloodstream of a person who eats large amounts of sucrose (table sugar). Cortisol comes from the adrenal glands, and high levels of cortisol can cause calcium deficiencies and osteoporosis. This is why doctors are more hesitant to prescribe corticosteroids due to the large amounts of bone loss that can occur. Since cortisol is a corticosteroid, one of the apparent links is that sugar can cause bone loss indirectly by creating cortisol.

In another study done by Dr. Yudkin, twenty-five teaspoons of table sugar was given to volunteers. When this was done, significant increases of calcium were seen in the volunteers' urine, suggesting that the sugar was leeching the body of its calcium and eliminating it. Something else to note in this study is that Dr. Yudkin noticed an even larger increase for individuals with a history of calcium oxalate kidney stones, suggesting that some people are more genetically prone to having a more pronounced reaction to sugar.¶¶ I would consider myself one of those people.

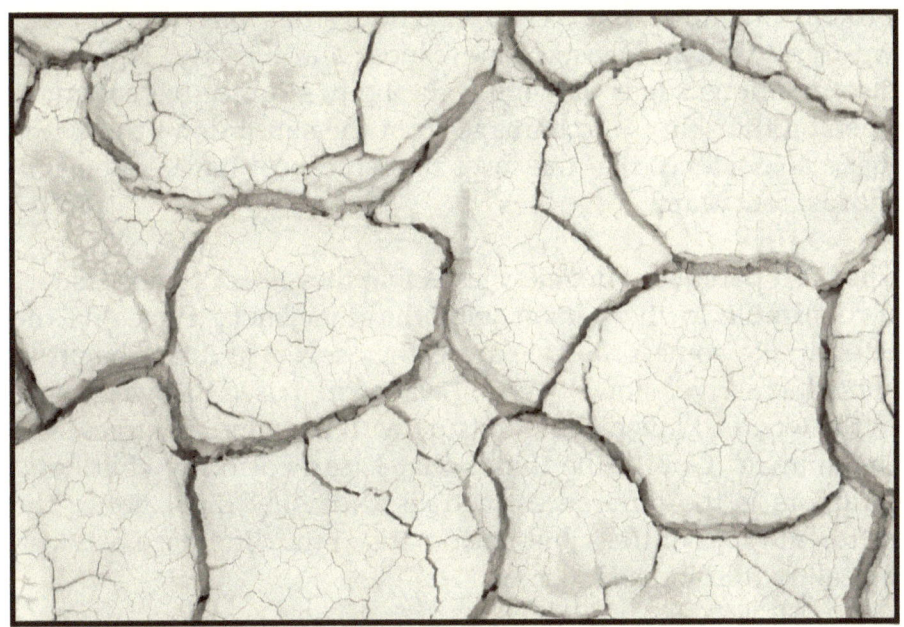

Illustration 7: Dry, cracked land, showing a deficiency of water.
There are numerous ways that our bodies show deficiencies
that we should pay attention to.

Another type of deficiency is dealing with your skin. Good, healthy skin needs collagen and elastin, which are protein fibers which keep the skin firm and less apt to wrinkle. There was a great article that came out recently on msnbc.msn.com called "Face Facts: Too Much Sugar Can Cause Wrinkles" by Karyn Repinski from *Prevention Magazine*.*** The article explained that the refined sugar in our bloodstream attaches itself to these

¶¶   www.healthy.net/scr/article.aspx?Id=1240,   Article   by
       Alan R. Gaby, MD, Excerpted from *Preventing and Reversing Osteoporosis*, Prima Publishing, 1996

***   http://www.msnbc.msn.com/id/21257751/ns/health-skin_
       and_beauty/t/face-facts-too-much-sugar-can-cause-
       wrinkles/#.TzCVWMWAHDU.

proteins in our skin, taking these proteins and turning them into harmful molecules in the body called cytokines, thus taking away the healthy proteins. They then do the same to the next protein, on and on like a chain reaction. After time, the skin that was once firm and elastic is now loose and wrinkly. The article also mentions sugar damaging the body's protective enzymes, opening the skin up to damage from the sun. I don't think it is just a coincidence that the cases of skin cancer have gone up in the last few years.

The hard part about deficiencies is that they are not immediately recognizable to the person with the deficiency. Typically, the effects take some time to expose themselves and can begin to show themselves slowly. When I was a kid, I used to love playing in the woods. I loved being outside with the wind, the trees, and the animals. One of the things that I learned in my childhood outdoors is the differences in trees. Not only did I notice the different types of trees, but I also noticed the difference between a healthy tree and a sick tree.

In looking at a live, healthy tree, a person can see that the tree is nice and strong. The bark doesn't have any holes in it, it has one steady color, there are no gaping or oozing wounds anywhere, and the bugs and birds generally leave the tree alone, besides building nests in it. A sick tree on the other hand usually has many discolorations in and on the bark, it has wounds here and there, and the birds and bugs are constantly attacking it, looking for a good home in the tree or a luscious meal.

I remember pulling the bark off of a sick tree and noticing the number of bugs underneath, eating away at the wood. The tree wasn't dead yet. In fact, it was still producing leaves and going through its normal cycles. In actuality, if you weren't paying attention, the tree would seem like a strong healthy tree. But underneath, it was a different story. The tree was only just beginning to break apart on the outside because it was being eaten from the inside out, usually from disease, lack of proper water, lack of nutrients, chemicals in the water, etc.

When we eat refined sugars, it is like putting little termites inside our body and letting them eat away. The removal of calcium and the collagen and elastin are only a few examples. And like the trees, oftentimes you won't notice until your body is already in pretty bad shape. Takeout: the removal of a substance needed for proper function and the second core effect of a diet high in refined sugars.

**

INFLAMMATION

I have a three-year-old daughter who is the cutest thing you ever saw. The problem is she knows it. But because she is so small and sounds like one of the munchkins from *The Wizard of Oz*, even if she is lying about why she broke your glasses, you still want to just pick her up because she's so cute. Everywhere we go, people are always commenting on how adorable she is.

But what is so shocking about my three-year-old daughter is the complete transformation that occurs when things don't go her way. When this happens, that cute little angel yells, pushes, and has at times thrown things. All of this, she says, is because her brother or sister made her do it. I tell you this because one of the things I've noticed is that when my three — year-old daughter loses her temper, her face really does turn red, and she gets hot and sweaty. I've seen her sitting on her bed, screaming at the top of her lungs, and looking like she was a thermometer with its round, red bulb about to pop. She becomes what I think is a good picture of "inflamed."

Inflammation is the last core effect that I want to discuss here and probably the most important. It is important not because it is any worse than the other core issues but because it is the one least talked about. Inflammation is the body's response to negative stimuli for healing purposes. It is how the body takes care of anything foreign that can harm it. It is usually characterized as having redness, swelling, heat, and pain. Think back to a time that you had a cut. What immediately happened to the area around the cut? It generally became red and swollen. This is because there is more blood that has been pushed into that area. More blood allows for the white blood cells to immediately attack any germs that have entered. More blood means more heat, which makes it harder for germs to live and reproduce (viruses and bacteria can multiply at extremely rapid rates.). The increased blood flow also allows the needed resources to stop the bleeding and to begin the process of repairing the skin. It is quite a large list of things that need to happen at the right time, order, and in the right quantities so we don't die from little cuts and bruises. The amazing thing is that it all happens on its own without our direction!

What about something bigger, maybe a time when you got a fever from an overgrowth of bacteria or viruses in your body. Your body's blood temperature rose (heat), your skin got flushed (redness), your glands began to swell (swelling), and you started to feel bad (pain). The body was actively fighting off the infection, and you were feeling the effects. It is important to speak of it this way (that the body was fighting off the infection) because many people today seem to have an image that the inflammatory response *is* the illness. With this, they take all kinds of medication to make the fever go away when it could help the body heal faster. I'm not saying that you should not take medication when you have a fever. High fevers can be very dangerous and one should always be very careful and should consult your physician on individual cases. What I am saying, though, is that we have a built-in illness fighter that we should all be aware of that can work for us. The body is an extremely intelligent and complex machine and its system of protection, the inflammatory response, is our friend . . . with one exception.

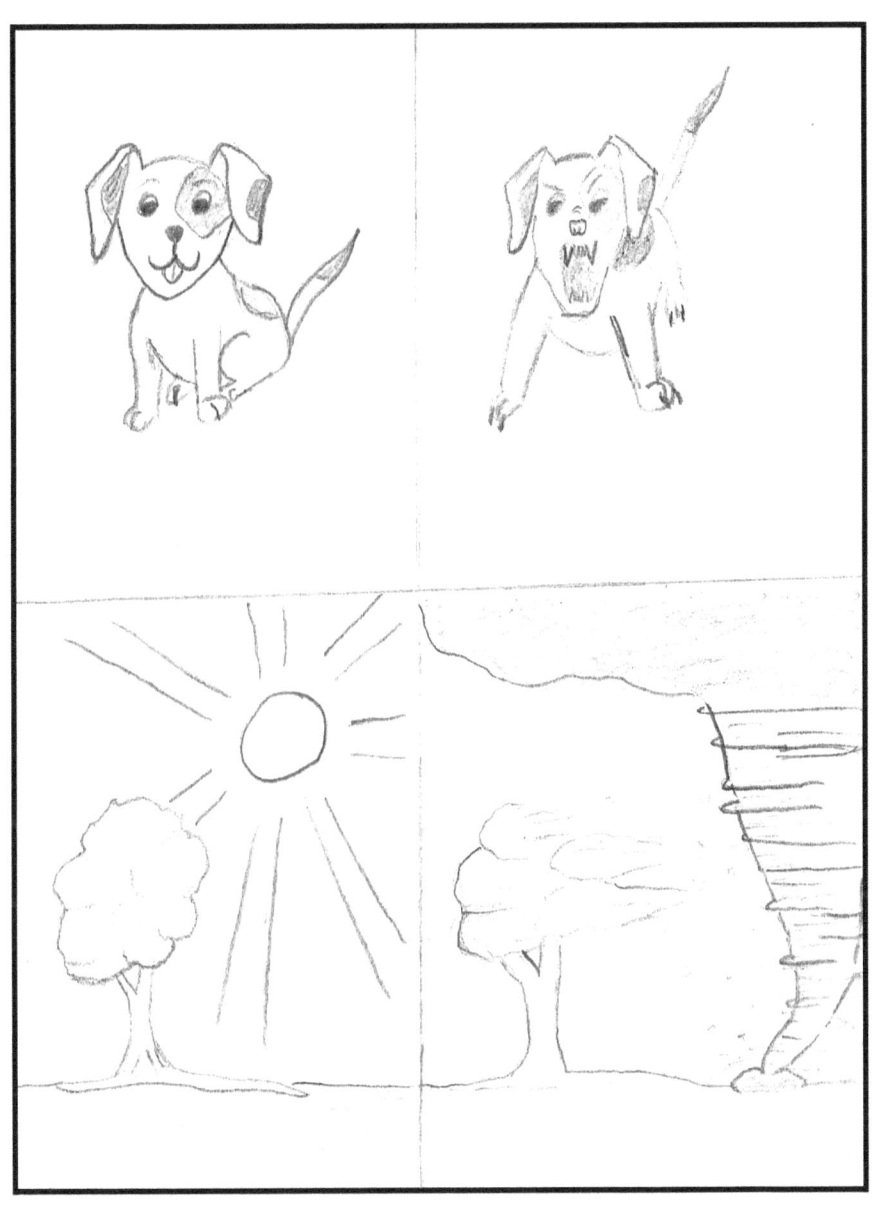

Illustration 8: An image of homeostasis vs. inflammation

I like analogies because it gives you a mental picture of something that is more complicated. In looking at how sugar affects our natural immune system, let me give you an analogy. The inflammatory system can be compared to a cat in a room. The cat loves to relax and lay around. It is calm and peaceful. But when there is a mouse in the room, it is the cat's automatic instinct to become heated, focused, and energized in order to hunt, catch, and kill the mouse. Then, once the mouse is dead, the cat lies down and takes another nap. Simply stated, this is just like the body's inflammatory response.

But what would happen to the cat in the room if it were forced to stay awake and chase mice 24/7 for days in a row? He definitely would not be functioning at his best. Most likely, the cat would become frazzled, jittery, and probably begin to pounce on anything that moves, including other cats or even its owner because it is so exhausted and confused. Eventually, the cat is going to pass out and maybe even die from overstimulation and exhaustion. Imagine if my three-year-old daughter had a temper tantrum constantly without ceasing. She would wear herself out.

When our immune system is triggered too often or over stimulated, the body's organs and tissues can become damaged. In fact, there is growing research that is linking inflammation as the underlying cause of most chronic diseases today—asthma, diabetes, lupus, arthritis, osteoporosis, periodontal disease, cardiovascular disease, high cholesterol, obesity, strokes, cancer, etc. I don't know if that sunk in, but that is a huge statement that I just made. The Center for Disease Control (CDC) states that chronic diseases account for 70% of all deaths in the U.S. (1.7 million people per year).[†††] That is equivalent to the entire population of the city of Philadelphia dying each year. The CDC also says that as of 2005, close to one out of every two people suffered from at least one chronic disease.

[†††]   Taken from http://www.cdc.gov/chronicdisease/overview/index.htm

In an article by Garry Egger, PhD, MPH entitled "In Search of a Germ Theory Equivalent for Chronic Disease," he says that "a form of low-grade systemic and chronic inflammation (metaflammation) [has been] linked to inducers (broadly termed anthropogens) associated with modern man-made environments and lifestyles, [which] suggests an underlying basis for chronic disease that could provide a twenty-first century equivalent of the germ theory."[‡‡‡] That was quite a mouthful. To put that in layman's terms, Mr. Egger is simply saying that our environment and lifestyle are causing constant inflammation within the body that is in turn causing our chronic diseases today. What is interesting is how he is saying that this finding will be as important as the discovery of germs, it is that important to our health!

So what are the main causes of inflammation? Dr. Duke Johnson, in his book *The Optimal Health Revolution,* says that the four largest causes of inflammation are pollution, high cholesterol intake, trans fatty acids, and (you guessed it) too many simple sugars.[§§§] I could spend a lot of time on the other three sources of inflammation, but as we are discussing sugar, I want to focus mainly on it. However, I do feel that it is just as important for each person to focus attention on these other three areas as well. Pollutants on our lives generally come from the air we breathe and the water we drink. So air purifiers and water treatment systems are essential today in our highly industrialized and chemical-laden environments. In terms of the high cholesterol and the eating of trans fatty acids, I'll just put it this way: God did not create trans fatty acids; He created fruits, vegetables, nuts, and meat-producing animals.

But what about sugar? Why is it considered one of the top four causes of inflammation? There are basically four markers, or indicators, that doctors use today to measure inflammation in

---

[‡‡‡]   Taken from http://www.cdc.gov/pcd/issues/2012/11_0301. htm

[§§§]   *The Optimal Health Revolution,* by Dr. Duke Johnson, MD. Benbella Books, Inc., 2008. pp. 42-43

a person's body.¶¶¶ Recent studies show that these markers are elevated when a person eats refined sugars. **** For one, as we've discussed, a steady diet of refined sugar causes an increase in the insulin levels in the body. One of the things that this increased insulin does is create an imbalance in what are called eicosanoids. These are hormones in the body that maintain healthy levels of inflammation. When the insulin level is high an imbalance occurs, causing inflammation which can be detected by one or more of the four markers. ††††

It is not healthy for the human body to be inflamed all the time. Think of all the — itis's that get regularly diagnosed today: gastritis, tonsillitis, sinusitis, colitis, arthritis, tendonitis, etc. The suffix itis literally means, "the inflammation of . . ." So, for example, if you have tendonitis you have inflammation of the tendons. Furthermore, if you have tonsillitis you have the inflammation of the tonsils. With all of the — itis's being diagnosed today, we can see how inflammation can be an underlying cause of most illnesses today. Oftentimes, we don't really even notice it at first. However, just like gold — plated jewelry, the sweatier you get and the more you expose it to chemicals like pool water, the quicker the gold plating wears away, exposing the metal underneath.

¶¶¶   C-reactive protein (CRP), haptoglobin, erythrocyte sedimentation rate (ESR), and transferrin

****   http://mpkb.org/home/pathogenesis/epidemiology

††††   "Inflammation" by Dr. Marcelle Pick, OB/GYN NP http://www.womentowomen.com/inflammation/causes.aspx

After several years in the military, where deployment to various locations in training and other operations prevented me from properly caring for my teeth, I started seeing a decline in my dental health. I began getting toothaches, my gums bled whenever I would floss or brush too hard, and discolorations cropped up on my teeth. In order to prevent further decay, I started using (mouthwash) religiously, flossed two to three times a day, and upped my brushing to three or four times a day. Despite my extensive efforts, my tooth issues continued, and I started consulting the Internet for home remedies that might work where modern dental technology had failed.

While surfing the Internet, I came across some startling articles discussing the link between diet and tooth decay. In these articles, various nutritionists compared the state of dental health in the U.S. and Western Europe to indigenous communities throughout the world which lacked even the most basic dental health technology. To my surprise, it appeared that these Third World communities enjoyed far better dental health than us here in the West despite the lack of dentistry or even toothbrushes, all because of their diet. Specifically, these indigenous people ate no refined sugar and consumed a much higher proportion of nutritionally dense, unprocessed, whole foods, resulting in strong teeth and robust health. According to these Internet articles, our consumption of sugar and other highly processed foods is a huge factor in our dental problems and the massive growth in obesity, diabetes, and heart disease in the West.

Testing that theory, I virtually eliminated refined sugar from my diet and began replacing sugary and processed foods with leafy greens, fruit, cod liver oil, and pastured meat and dairy, and within a few months, my tooth problems had evaporated. My gums stopped bleeding, the discolored spots began whitening, and I simply felt better. In an era of advanced medicine, too many Americans have forgotten that the easiest and simplest way to better health comes from what you eat. I would recommend to anyone experiencing health issues to begin by reducing one of the plagues of modern society: sugar.

Pat (Patrick)
Atlanta, GA

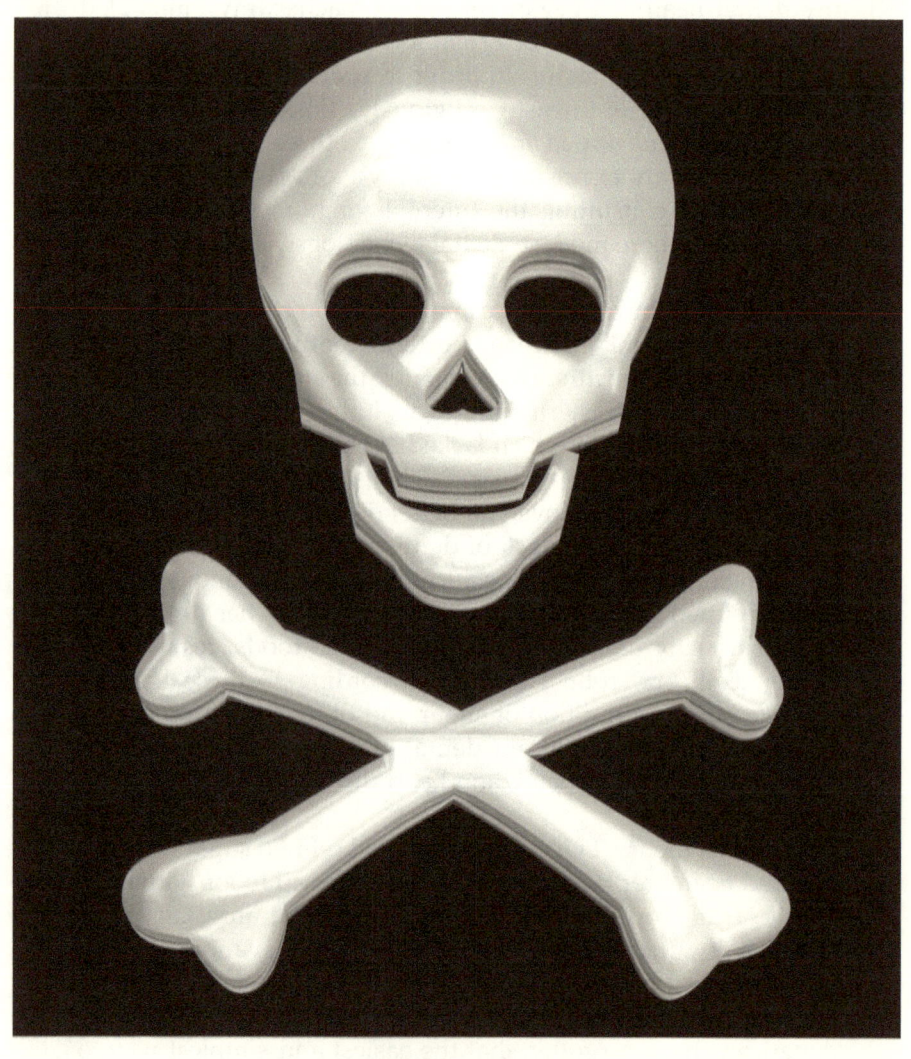

Illustration 9: The skull and crossbones, used to signify
that something is poisonous or dangerous.

Chapter 5: Sugar—Is It a Poison?

"It is not about the calories . . . It has nothing to do with the calories. It's a poison by itself."[‡‡‡‡]

Robert Lustig, in his speech "Sugar: The Bitter Truth"

(Lustig is a pediatric hormone disorders specialist and expert in childhood obesity at the University of California, San Francisco, School of Medicine)

I have referred to sugar as a poison numerous times already and have tried to do as thorough of a job as I could in explaining how sugar is negatively affecting our health. But is sugar a poison? If by sugar, you are referring to unrefined sugars, the answer is overwhelmingly no. Sugar is essential to life. However, as we are referring to refined sugars, that is another matter.

The dictionary describes a poison as:

"A substance that can kill, injure, or impair an organism by means of its chemical action."[§§§§]

Furthermore, a chemical is defined as:

"A substance that is created from or by a chemical process (or reaction) . . ."[¶¶¶¶]

[‡‡‡] "I got this off of a speech that I heard by Dr. Lustig on YouTube called *Sugar: The Bitter Truth.* But Dr. Robert Lustig has written a great book called *Fat Chance: The Bitter Truth About Sugar.*

[§§§§] *Merriam-Webster's School Dictionary*, printed by Merriam-Webster Inc, 2004. p. 742

[¶¶¶¶] *Merriam-Webster's School Dictionary*, printed by Merriam-Webster Inc, 2004. p. 160

With this in mind, let's take a look at how sugar is made from sugarcane to see if any chemical processes were involved. We'll let the process itself expose whether or not it is a chemical . . .

I'm sorry for the scientific terms in this description, but I used them to prove the point.

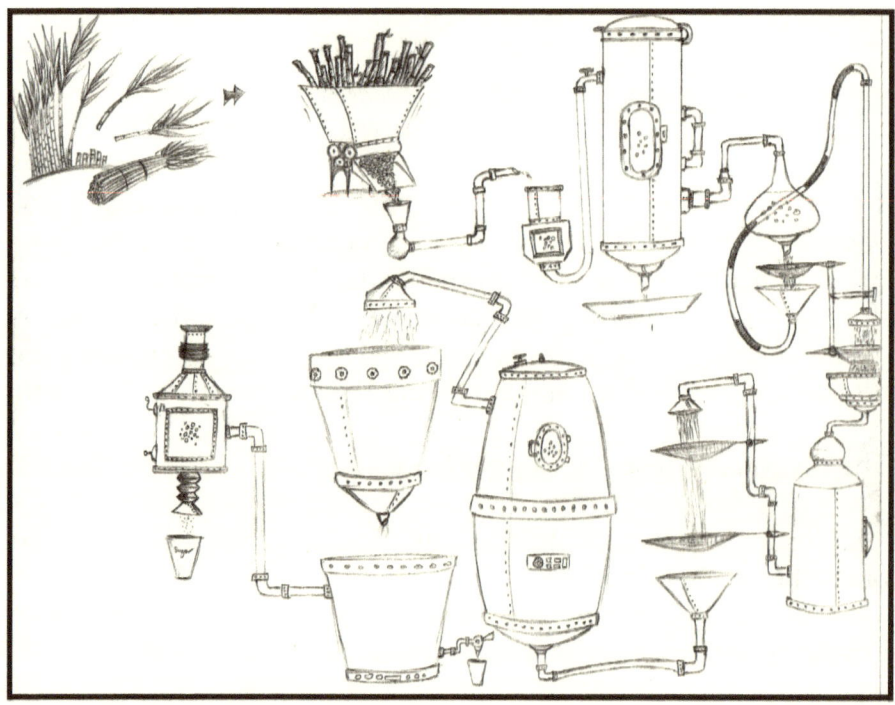

Illustration 10: Front cover image by Tim Kasa.
The process of making sugar.

Once the juice is extracted from the sugarcane, sulfur dioxide vapors are passed through the juice in a process called sulphitation (chemical reaction #1) to leach the juice (i.e. pull out the juice from the solid material). Then the leached juice is added to a vat that has water mixed with powdered lime. This mixture is then stirred for about six hours so that the mixture goes through a process called alkalization (chemical reaction #2).

Once this is completed, it goes into a clarifier tank where it sits. In the tank, the impurities settle to the bottom while the juice is left on top. After the impurities (resembling mud) are filtered out, the remaining juice is then placed in large tanks called evaporators and boiled to evaporate most of the water in the juice.

Once this is done, the remaining juice is again placed in tanks to clarify. The remaining sediment floats to the top and is skimmed off. By now what was juice has become a thick, brown syrup. Microscopic sucrose crystals suspended in alcohol are then added to this syrup. This solution binds to the sugar (chemical reaction #3) in the syrup to draw it out. Again, the syrup is boiled in large vacuum tanks to form sugar crystals as the water continues to boil away. Once there is a very thick brown paste, it goes into high-speed centrifugal machines that separate the crystals from the uncrystalized syrup. This syrup is molasses, which is drained out while it spins. Water is then sprayed on the crystals and drained out as well, leaving only the washed, raw sugar crystals.

That is how sucrose is made from sugarcane. I counted three chemical reactions that took place in that process. But before we go further, let's also take a look at how high fructose corn syrup is made . . .

High fructose corn syrup starts out as corn starch. This starch is then mixed with water and a bacterial enzyme that breaks the starch down (chemical reaction#1). Add another fungal enzyme which breaks the molecules down into glucose molecules (chemical reaction #2) and you now have corn syrup. Add another bacterial enzyme and about half of the glucose is converted (chemical reaction #3) into fructose. This is now high fructose corn syrup.[*****]

So is refined sugar a chemical—"a substance created from a chemical process . . . ?" Based on the definition above, I would

---

[*****] diabeteshealth.com/read/2011/«/how-high-fructose-corn-syrup-hfcs-is-made

say the answer is yes. It started out as one thing and became something different through chemical processes.

But more important is the second reason why it is a poison, which is the way it reacts in the body. Just like the definition says above, refined sugar is able to "kill, injure, or impair." This whole book is focusing on this aspect of sugar. But something to reiterate here is that sugar doesn't kill immediately for most people. It is a slow, degrading type of death, much like rust on a bridge.

When I was in school, I learned about the art of comparison to study chemicals in science. In general, we can't witness the actual chemical reaction first hand because it happens at the molecular level. I don't know about you, but I can't see things that small. However, when a chemical reaction does occur, we can notice it through its byproducts. For instance, if there is a reaction in a jar when I mix two chemicals, we might feel heat when there was no heat there before. You might also see a change in color or a thickening or thinning of the substance. There might be bubbles or even fire. Along these same lines, when studying how different chemicals work together, the different reactions are written down and called properties. So if chemical A always produces bubbles when chemical B is added to it, that is one of chemical B's properties. Now, if chemical C is added to chemical A and also creates bubbles, scientists would say that chemical C is similar in its chemical properties as chemical B. So the chemicals are rated similar by the reactions/properties. When dealing with sugar, we can compare it to the drug heroin in terms of how the body reacts to both substances.

For one thing, both heroin and sugar affect the pleasure portion of the brain to make us "feel" good. When heroin enters the body, it is immediately absorbed and bathes the pleasure centers of the brain, giving us that extreme high. Sugar does the same thing, just not as intensely. We've all had a sugar high—they don't call it a sugar "high" for nothing. It is not uncommon to see heroin addicts consuming large amounts of sugar when they are not high on heroin. They are trying to fight off the deep lows they feel from not having the heroin in their system. Sugar helps calm the cravings.

Another similarity between the drug heroin and sugar is the addictiveness.[†††††] Once you've sampled heroin and felt the high, the lack of heroin in the system once it wears off brings upon an extreme low. What was once normal now feels like a low compared to the high we felt with the drug. Sugar also brings the same low after a high. We have all felt this as well. We call it "the crash." This is most often caused by low blood sugar as we've discussed before, but it is also due to having created an addiction in the pleasure portion of our brain. Kathleen DesMaisons, PhD asked some poignant questions in her book *The Sugar Addict's Total Recovery Program* that I believe let us answer the question for ourselves. Paraphrasing what she said, DesMaisons asked "Have you ever just tried to eat one piece of candy or cake? Has the number of packets of sugar you use in your coffee or tea decreased or increased over time? Have you ever said, 'I need some sugar for a quick pick-me-up?' Have you found yourself drinking more and more sugary drinks, energy sports drinks included? Do you ever just crave something sweet? Do you get really cranky when you haven't had something sugary for a couple of days?"[‡‡‡‡‡] My guess is that many of you said yes to at least one of these questions. That sounds like a dependency. Heroin and sugar both create a tolerance and dependence at the same time.

Again, much of this has to do with the fact that the high we feel is so great that it makes everything else seem bland. That is one of the reasons why so many people think naturally created foods like vegetables, fruits, and grains are not flavorful; it is because they eat so much sugar that their taste buds are desensitized, making the other foods seem flavorless. Just like heroin addicts are desensitized to the pleasures of life, sugar addicts are

---

[†††††]   for a good article on this, see Dr. Frank Lipman's article at http://www.drfranklipman.com/are-you-a-sugar-addict.

[‡‡‡‡‡]   DesMaisons, Kathleen PhD, *The Sugar Addict's Total Recovery Program*

desensitized to taste. Miriam Vos, MD, MSPH, spoke about this in her book *The No-Diet Obesity Solution for Kids*. In her book, she commented on the fact that the more sugar you eat, the more you need to eat in order to taste the sugar. In fact, it happens so fast that by the time you finish eating that lollipop or cupcake, you can't taste the food anymore. The first bite is always the best.

I remember when I finally broke my addiction to sugar. It was as though foods all of a sudden had taste. Spinach, broccoli, sugar-free peanut butter . . . they all started to seem rich in flavor that they lacked before. I also noticed that foods high in sugar now only tasted like sugar, nothing else.

Make no mistake; many of us in America are plain-old sugar junkies, hooked on the chemical of sugar that is harming us. Harvey Diamond said it well in his book called *Fit for Life: A New Beginning*, when he called refined sugar "a deadly and virulent poison."[§§§§§] I would have to agree.

[§§§§§] Fit for Life: A New Beginning — The Ultimate Diet and Health Plan. By Harvey Diamond

This (eating healthy) is a huge conviction in our lives, but I want to preface it that our conviction comes, not from a health or vanity perspective, but a spiritual perspective. It wasn't until the Lord convicted our hearts that our bodies are truly a temple of the living God did we make changes in nutrition and exercise that have stuck. We want to take care of our bodies and our children's bodies so that we can be as strong and healthy as possible, free from the burdens of disease and health issues, so that we can serve and glorify God without those stumbling blocks.

We aren't sugar-free in the sense that we do eat fruits and use honey, but we definitely try to avoid refined sugars, "dead" flour, and processed foods in general. Over the course of many years, we have slowly eliminated refined and processed foods, sticking to foods in their natural states and eating grains as unprocessed as possible or freshly milled.

We have seen huge improvements in the strength of our immune and digestive systems. I used to struggle with seasonal allergies, and I rarely (if ever) have any flare ups. No one in our family has had a need for allergy or any other kind of medication in recent years. We rarely have issues with colds or the flu; and if we start catching a virus, our immune systems have been strong enough to fight it off without the use of pharmaceuticals.

We strongly believe that this is possible because of our convictions with nutrition (not *diet*) and exercise. Our two young boys are certainly lively, energetic boys; but nutrition, adequate exercise, and Biblical discipline have resulted in children without attention issues or other health problems.

Ultimately all the glory goes to God. At any minute, He could see fit to humble us with some sort of problem that defies all our nutrition efforts. We do recognize that. However, we feel that in general, He blesses our efforts to honor Him by obeying the wisdom in His word regarding how to care for the bodies He has given us that are made in His image, eating the foods that He designed for them to use as fuel.

Scott and Christy
Cumming, GA

Did you know that . . .
Sugar can suppress the immune system.
Sugar can upset the body's mineral balance.
Sugar can contribute to hyperactivity, anxiety, depression, concentration difficulties, and crankiness in children.
Sugar can produce a significant rise in triglycerides.
Sugar can cause drowsiness and decreased activity in children.
Sugar can reduce helpful high density cholesterol (HDLs).
Sugar can promote an elevation of harmful cholesterol (LDLs).
Sugar can cause hypoglycemia.
Sugar contributes to a weakened defense against bacterial infection.
Sugar can cause kidney damage.
Sugar can increase the risk of coronary heart disease.
Sugar may lead to chromium deficiency.
Sugar can cause copper deficiency.
Sugar interferes with absorption of calcium and magnesium.
Sugar can increase fasting levels of blood glucose.
Sugar can promote tooth decay.
Sugar can produce an acidic stomach.
Sugar can raise adrenaline levels in children.
Sugar can lead to periodontal disease.
Sugar can speed the aging process, causing wrinkles and grey hair.
Sugar can increase total cholesterol.
Sugar can contribute to weight gain and obesity.
High intake of sugar increases the risk of Crohn's disease and ulcerative colitis.
Sugar can contribute to diabetes.
Sugar can contribute to osteoporosis.
Sugar can cause a decrease in insulin sensitivity.
Sugar leads to decreased glucose tolerance
Sugar can cause cardiovascular disease.

Continued on next page . . .

. . . continued from previous page.

Sugar can increase systolic blood pressure.
Sugar causes food allergies.
Sugar can cause free radical formation in the bloodstream.
Sugar can cause toxemia during pregnancy.
Sugar can contribute to eczema in children.
Sugar can overstress the pancreas, causing damage.
Sugar can cause atherosclerosis.
Sugar can compromise the lining of the capillaries.
Sugar can cause liver cells to divide, increasing the size of the liver.
Sugar can increase the amount of fat in the liver.
Sugar can increase kidney size and produce pathological changes in the kidney.
Sugar can cause depression.
Sugar can increase the body's fluid retention.
Sugar can cause hormonal imbalance.
Sugar can cause hypertension.
Sugar can cause headaches, including migraines.
Sugar can cause an increase in delta, alpha, and theta brain waves, which can alter the mind's ability to think clearly.
Sugar can increase blood platelet adhesiveness which increases risk of blood clots and strokes.
Sugar can increase insulin responses in those consuming high-sugar diets compared to low-sugar diets.
Sugar increases bacterial fermentation in the colon.

Source: www.nancyappleton.com

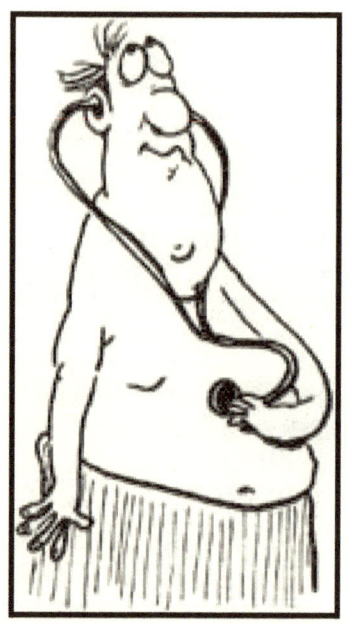

Illustration 11: Man listening to his own heartbeat. If you pay attention to your own body, most times it will tell you what is going on inside.

Chapter 6: The Other Effects of Sugar

"Diet is a significant factor in the risk of coronary heart disease (CHD), certain types of cancer, and strokes—the three leading causes of death in the United States; and responsible for over half of all deaths in 1994. Diet also plays a major role in the development of diabetes (the seventh leading cause of death), hypertension, and obesity. These six health conditions incur considerable medical expenses, lost work, disability, and premature deaths—much of it unnecessary, since a significant proportion of these conditions is believed to be preventable through improved diets."(24)

—United States Department of Agriculture Statistic[¶¶¶¶¶]

"Not only does eating too much sugar lead to obesity, diabetes, and tooth decay, it is also one of the biggest contributors to low energy and feelings of being overwhelmed—it has even been scientifically linked to depression."[******]

—Dr. Frank Lipman

Beep . . . beep . . . beep . . . beep . . . beep . . . beep . . . BAM! Beep . . . beep . . . beep . . . BAM! You just hit the snooze button; probably the third or fourth time this morning. You need to get up or else you are going to be late . . . but you are soooo tired . . . just five more minutes! You force yourself to get up, doing the morning shuffle to the bathroom, running into walls and grunting to the kids to wake up. You get in the shower and feel a bit revived from the warm water running over your face. You step out of the shower and feel clearer-minded from the fresh air only to look at the clock on the wall and realize that you are late! OH, NO! Gotta get going! You hurry up the kids. No time for bacon, eggs, and toast this morning (like you have it *any* morning). You blurt out

---

[¶¶¶¶¶]   http://www.ers.usda.gov/publications/aib750

[******]   "Dr. Frank Lipman, M. D. has a great website (www.drfranklipman.com) and has written two books, *Total Renewal: 7 Key Steps to Resilience, Vitality and Long Term Health and Revive: Stop Feeling Spent and Start Living Again*".

to the kids among their requests for food, "Grab a cinnamon roll or sugar tart! Wait! On second thought, we'll stop at the drive through." You think, "We'll just get some doughnuts and orange juice." You pull everyone together, and you head out the door.

Once the kids are dropped off at school, you race to work and get there just in time for your morning meeting. It is a busy and trying meeting; so afterward, you feel the need for a pick-me-up. You stop by the vending machines and get a soda and a bag of chips. You continue on with your day when before you know it, it is lunch time and you are starving again! You didn't have anything nutritious for breakfast or snack, and you're thinking you should eat something healthy, but in your hurry this morning, you forgot to pack a lunch. With not much time, and let's face it not much money, you decide to pick up a few cheap tacos and burritos from the local fast food restaurant. And for dessert... sopapillas — tortilla chips with honey, chocolate syrup, and cinnamon! Mmm!

Your afternoon is drudgery because you can't seem to get any energy. You're constantly feeling tired after lunch. Soon it is time to get home for the kids. You rush to the car and are on your way. On the road, you start thinking "what are we going to have for dinner?" You start imagining the effort it will take and the mess you will make putting together something healthy and nutritious. "No, something fast sounds better." You stop at the grocery on the way home and pick up a few frozen pizzas, some hotdogs, and a few packs of macaroni and cheese. The kids will love it! And they do. And for dessert . . . ice cream!

Does this sound a bit familiar? It should because this is how many of us function at least five out of seven days of the week. With the relatively new technologies of TV, computers, and cell phones that were supposed to make our lives easier and more relaxed, we now have so many more inputs into our lives that make us feel overwhelmed with things to do. Not to mention that work hours have increased, and many men and women today are performing the job of a parent alone. We all feel very busy as a society. Unfortunately, in the name of convenience the idea of a good diet goes neglected.

In today's society, it is much cheaper and easier to eat quick-and-easy, ready-made meals with very little nutritional value and lots of preservatives. On top of that, we feel the need to have something sugary with every meal, almost feeling that a meal is not complete without it. We crave for our sugar tarts, sugary cereals, doughnuts, candy bars, cookies, pies, and cakes. But what is really going on here? Why is this important enough to write a whole book about sugar? We've already been discussing refined sugar and its bad effects on our lives. In general, I think most people already know the majority of what I've discussed anyway. What I really want is for you to think about how much refined sugar is affecting your own personal life. Again, this is not an individual diagnosis and should not take the place of your physician's professional counsel. But I do want to get you asking yourself, "Is sugar really affecting me and how?"

Let's take a close up look at some of the chronic "diseases"†††††† that people are suffering from today. I'm not covering all chronic diseases (and there are plenty), just some of the more common ones. The main purpose is to define each disease and show you how sugar can either cause or affect the disease. I also want to point out how interrelated almost all of these diseases really are. For instance, eczema is a result of the inflammatory response of the body. If it is happening on the skin that is visible, what do you think is happening beneath the skin? Eczema could be a good early indicator of other issues going on. Diabetes is another example. The connection between diabetes and heart disease has today been well established and will be discussed below.

***

---

†††††† I put "diseases" in quotations because many of the diseases under the heading of chronic illness are simply a set of symptoms with no specific cause, like you would have with an infectious disease. In most cases, chronic diseases are all related, which is why many people suffer from more than one at a time.

Tooth Decay

> *"Inflammation is a common link between periodontal diseases and diabetes."*[††††††]

We've all been told that eating lots of food with sugar will cause tooth decay. But have you ever wondered how? Not only is sugar acidic, promoting the plaque and gingivitis that our dentists all tell us about; but sugar also robs the body of its minerals, just like it does to heroin addicts, just not as rapidly. We've already discussed calcium and how sugar robs this mineral from the teeth and bones.[§§§§§§] But just to reiterate, if your diet is high in sugar, the sugar robs all the available calcium in the food you eat and your body will actually remove what was already there in your bones for use. Once the teeth and bones are weak, infections and disease are more able to infest. This includes tooth decay but is not limited to it.

This is a good example of both deficiency and burnout. But if this is happening to your teeth, think of what else could be going on inside your body at the same time. Oftentimes, one symptom is a good indicator of something else going on. In this case, tooth decay or gum disease can be an indicator of heart disease. If it causes issues with your teeth, do you think it leaves the rest of the body alone? It is not surprising that gum disease is a real issue with people who have diabetes. An article put out by the Journal of American Dental Association in 2006 noted that teenagers with type 1 diabetes were five time more likely to have gum disease than if they didn't have diabetes. It also mentioned that people with type 2 diabetes were three times more likely to have gum disease than if

---

[††††††]   *Periodontal disease and diabetes: A two-way street* by Brian L. Mealey, DDS, MS. (pgs 30 & 31) posted on http://www.ada.org/sections/professionalResources/pdfs/Perio_diabetes.pdf and originally included in the Journal of American Dental Association, Vol. 137, Oct 2006.

[§§§§§§]   For more information, see chapter 4 on deficiency.

they didn't have diabetes.¶¶¶¶¶¶ Gum disease and cavities can be a great early warning system for diabetes and heart disease. We will discuss further the link between diabetes and heart disease below. But overall, if we pay attention to our bodies and notice the small aches, itches, twitches, or simple changes, we oftentimes can make changes to help prevent the larger issues from emerging which can drastically affect or even shorten our lives.

***

Obesity

"During the past 20 years, there has been a dramatic increase in obesity in the United States and rates remain high. More than one-third of U.S. adults (35.7%) and approximately 17% (or 12.5 million) of children and adolescents aged 2-19 years are obese."

Source: The Center for Disease Control and Prevention (CDC)
at http://www.cdc.gov/obesity/data/facts.html.

" . . . eating fructose (high fructose corn syrup, for example) causes far more accumulation of abdominal fat—the most dangerous kind—than other forms of sugar, even if the same number of calories is consumed."

The Sugar Fix: The High Fructose Fallout
That Is Making You Fat and Sick by Richard J. Johnson,
MD, and Timothy Gower*******

In 1985, the number of obese individuals in the U.S. was less than 10% of the population with only six states having a maximum of 14% as obese. (For those who are not aware, obesity is defined as having a body mass index (BMI) of 30 or greater.††††††††) In 2010, only twenty-five years later, this number has doubled with over

---

¶¶¶¶¶¶ Periodontal disease and diabetes: A two-way street by Brian L. Mealey, DDS, MS. (pgs 27)

******* *The Sugar Fix: The High Fructose Fallout That Is Making You Fat and Sick* by Richard J. Johnson, Rodale Inc. ©2008, pp. 7-8.

†††††††† To calculate the body mass index (BMI), take your weight in pounds, multiply it by 703 and divide the total by your height

20% of the population being obese. Twelve of our states have 30% or more of its people obese and the remaining states have over 20%. Colorado has the lowest rate of obesity with only 21%. *Only 21%*, that is one out of every five people. That is a huge increase from 1985.[#######]

Obesity is one of those topics that is highly discussed but also highly sensitive. With all of the weight-loss gimmicks and miracle pills, it can seem to fog up our vision of the truth about how to be healthy. So many people are tired of trying fad diet after fad diet. How many times have you gone on a diet, lost weight, and then gained more back? Well, you can rest easy. I am not going to make any claims on having the patent to weight loss for every individual. My own personal belief is that there are too many factors in each person's body to make a blanket claim that applies to everyone. It is like my kids. Every one of them has a different personality and therefore requires a different approach to parenting. My oldest, for example, has never required any harsh punishment.

She loves harmony and has always hated to have Mom and Dad be upset with her. So when she did something she shouldn't have, all we had to do was talk about it and express our displeasure. If it was bad enough, we'd take away a privilege or a toy for a while. My second daughter, on the other hand, is more independent and conflict-oriented. In fact, she seems to thrive on conflict. Sometimes, I think she does things just because I tell her not to. Punishment is a regular thing in her life so much so that we've had to really focus on making sure we give her plenty of love throughout the day to offset the discipline. This is a great example of the differences in people. Just like my two girls are very different in personality; all people are different when it comes to their genetics and what it will take to live a healthy lifestyle.

---

in inches squared, e.g., 150 lbs × 703 / 69″ × 69″ = a BMI of 22.1487

[#######] Centers for Disease Control and Prevention, U.S. Obesity Trends: http://www.cdc.gov/obesity/data/trends.HTML

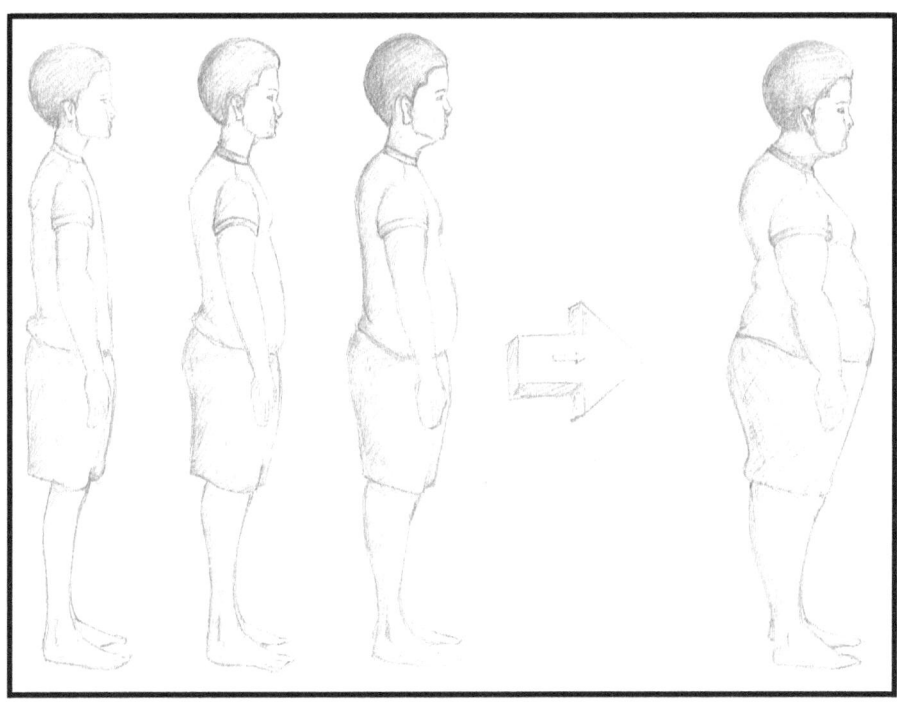

Illustration 12: Being unhealthy is not an overnight thing; it occurs over time.
You need to make lifestyle changes to be healthy and lose weight,
not go on temporary diets. Drawing by Tim Kasa.

Even though our bodies are different, the knowledge of how to have a healthy and fit body is available if you are willing to look for it. What is even more important is that once you find the knowledge, you have to be willing to follow it because oftentimes it takes discipline and change. It is just as the Bible says, "Seek and ye shall find, knock and the door shall be opened for you." But never forget, you still have to walk through the door. Many people are simply looking for that microwave solution. They want the miracle pill, the *one* thing they can do to solve all of their woes. Unfortunately, it usually takes more than one life change to reach the status of "healthy." If you would like to lose weight, a great place to start is researching your genetics. There are genetic tests today that determine your body type—how you process different types of foods, what is the best balance of foods, and how much exercise is required for you to stay fit. It is a quick and easy test. All you have to do is rub a cotton swab on the inside of your cheek and send it in to a laboratory to be analyzed. Scientists have now found the genes that can define a person's body type. Once you find out your body type, you can better put together a health plan that works specifically for you.

Another change to make would be to begin a regular habit of exercise, whether it be through certain activities like sports or physical hobbies or at the gym, just make sure your heart rate is up and that you are sweating. I know sweating can be uncomfortable, but so is being in a hospital bed having bypass surgery. Exercise is the hardest and most uncomfortable when your body is not used to it. Once you get used to it, it is not that hard, and you feel so much better for having done it.

The last area to change, of course is your diet. You had to know that was coming since this is a book about sugar. Diet and nutrition is so crucial, though, and where the genetics testing will come in handy. This testing will tell you what the proper diet is for your body type as well as how much and what type of exercise will work best. But it is all geared around your particular body type.

Even with all of these body type differences, one constant remains, that refined sugar is unhealthy and should be removed or severely restricted from the diet. There is more to it than just being a good idea. Sugar is also a major factor in obesity. In a study completed by the American Society for Nutrition, they have concluded that in just the last ten years, the consumption of sugar-sweetened beverages, like soda and energy drinks, has gone up. They also found that sugar-sweetened drinks are the number one source of beverage calories and a considerable source of the daily calories. This study also directly linked this sugar intake with obesity and type 2 diabetes saying that the consumption of sugar-sweetened drinks are the highest among subgroups such as lower income families and African Americans, which are at the greatest risk of obesity and type 2 diabetes.[§§§§§§§]

[§§§§§§§]   *The American Journal of Clinical Nutrition,* "Increasing Consumption of Sugar-Sweetened Beverages among U.S. Adults: 1988-1994 to

As I mentioned in chapter four, eating refined sugar is like pouring jet fuel into the engine of your car. When there is so much sugar forced into the bloodstream, the body is forced to deal with it. And how does our body handle all of the excess fuel that surges into the bloodstream? It stores it as extra fat. This is interesting because in the early part of the 1980's the Surgeon General of the United States informed America that the nation was too fat and that we as a nation needed to cut out the high fatty foods thinking that this would slim down the nation. Of course the manufacturing companies jumped on the bandwagon and got rid of the fat in their foods. But guess what they replaced the fat with . . . sugar! And now, according to the Center for Disease Control, over twenty years later, obesity has not decreased, but increased 15 to 20%. (Again, "obesity" being defined as having a body mass index of 30 or over *or* a body fat percentage of around 25% to 30%)¶¶¶¶¶¶¶

I believe many physicians would agree that we as a society are overweight partially due to the large amounts of sugar and simple carbohydrates (which turn to sugar) in our diets. If people would simply cut out sodas, sugary coffees, ice cream, candy bars, and cakes, we would all notice a significant difference. We live in one of the most prosperous nations in the world, yet over 60% of our society suffers from obesity. There is something wrong with that. But what is really alarming is how obese our children are getting. In the last twenty years, the rate of obesity in children and adolescents has doubled! When I see a child no older than five already huffing and puffing from going up the stairs or throwing the ball around, I fear for the child. Not only is the child's health at stake, but so is his/her self-esteem. We live in a society that is cruel to people who struggle with their weight.

But why is sugar so hard to turn away? Part of this issue with sugars is that it appeals to our self-centered natures. When dealing with stress or any kind of physical or emotional pain, eating is used by many as a means of comfort and self-pity. And what do most people crave when they are upset? Sugar or

---

1999-2004": http://www.ajcn.org/content/89/1/372.abstract.
¶¶¶¶¶¶¶ See the footnote on previous page about calculating BMI.

simple carbohydrates which turns to sugar quickly in the body. Why not choose a salad, fruits, or vegetables to eat when we are depressed? It would be a lot healthier. Why is it always the sweets? Because sugar is a drug and it is *very* addictive. This is something you will notice when you take *The Dare*. Depending on how much sugar you currently eat and how addicted to it you are, you will go through withdrawal. Many of you will become grumpy and a little unpleasant to be around. Some of you will get headaches and massive cravings. It won't be as bad as if you were a recovering heroin addict or an alcoholic, but in reality you will suffer from withdrawal. One of my dear friends calls herself a "dry alcoholic," referring to her love of sweets and her physical addiction. It is the same with all of us; when we break the habit, it will be like getting sober, just not nearly as bad. And of course, how you feel once you've broken the addiction is worth the effort!

Another reason why sugar is hard to turn away is the psychological addiction. Sugar tastes and feels good. Oftentimes, we don't really want to cut it out of our diets and feel angry at anyone who might imply that we should. I've had people laugh at me and even get belligerent when they discovered my dietary discipline. I was the same way. When I made my first attempt at *The Dare* and cut sugar from my diet, I went around with a storm cloud over my head. I felt like I was being punished by not being able to eat sugary foods. I craved sugar. And when I was hungry and saw other people eating sugar, I would usually have a grown-up temper tantrum — that is when you take out your anger on other people by pouting and fussing. I cannot apologize enough to my wife for having made her go through that. But the good news is that it didn't last forever. And today, though my mind sometimes tells me that I want that cookie or piece of cake, if I ever give in and eat it, it never tastes as good as my mind remembers. It really only has one flavor, sugar. And once you are actually free from the bondage of sugar, you realize there is much more to taste.

In summary, taking *The Dare* and cutting out or severely limiting refined sugar from your diet can only add benefit to what you are already doing. If you are overweight or obese, let me highly encourage you to take *The Dare* for yourself and get free from the bondage of sugary foods.

***

Depression/Bipolar Disorder/ Psychosis/Unclear Thinking/Low Energy

"I have found in my practice that how a person metabolizes not only simple sugars and complex carbs but also proteins and fats is a crucial factor in as many as three out of every five cases of depression (that's 60 out of every 100 cases, or 60%!)."

Depression-Free for Life by Gabriel Cousens, MD

"In my own clinical experience, mild to moderate depression is closely linked to diet. High sugar consumption goes hand-in-hand with what is generally labeled as depression."

The Sugar Addict's Total Recovery Program by Kathleen DesMaisons, PhD

"According to Rita Elkins, MH, in Solving the Depression Puzzle, "We have become obsessed with sugar, not fully recognizing what excessive sugar consumption not only does to the body, but also to the mind . . . (Rita Elkins) cites studies by Richard Wurtman, MD, and Judith Wurtman, PhD, of MIT (Richard Wurtman is the co-author of The Serotonin Solution), who found that sugar and starch in carbohydrates temporarily boost serotonin levels, which would account for the carbohydrate cravings in people who are prone to depression. Additionally, depressed people are drawn to sugar and fat combinations such as those found in cookies and chocolate."(30)

Living Well with Depression and Bipolar Disorder by John McManamy

Depression is another controversial topic, just like obesity. And just like with the debate on obesity, there are many opinions about depression as well. For many, depression is a disease that can be treated with pharmaceuticals. To others, depression is a genetic trait, passed down from one's parents and grandparents. For others, depression is more a residual of one's childhood that has yet to be dealt with. An example of this would be an adult who is still suffering from habits created from early child abuse or abandonment. And lastly, there are those who see depression as simply an issue of personality, a person who has a more self-focused perspective on life.

But no matter what the source of depression, when it comes to diet, there have been some very interesting findings that link a person's mental state and a diet that is high in sugar. Gabriel Cousens, MD, mentioned in his book *Depression-Free for Life*, that how a person metabolizes proteins and fats as well as simple sugars and carbohydrates plays a major part in at least three out of every five cases of depression. That is saying that in 60% of all of his cases, diet is affecting their depression . . . 60%! What these findings could also be saying is that a person's genetics might be playing a part in how much sugar and other foods are affecting them. This definitely makes it harder to narrow down symptoms in people, but it can be done. In my case, I am predisposed to blood-sugar issues because of the genes that were passed down to me by my parents. With this, I can attest that sugar does affect my moods significantly. Before I stopped eating refined sugar, I used to have large mood swings. I would get into real deep lows that would sometimes last weeks. I would have my highs too. But when I cut out sugar, one of the things I noticed was that my moods stayed steady. I still have my normal ups and downs, but they never feel very low, and they don't last very long.******** Of course, I have other tools to combat the lows like exercise, reading positive books, listening to positive music, and getting around positive people. But taking out the sugar made it a lot easier to do all of these other things.

******** Let me also strongly recommend a strong spiritual life as well. A life without a purpose is like a ship without a rudder, just floating with the tide and moving wherever the next storm takes them.

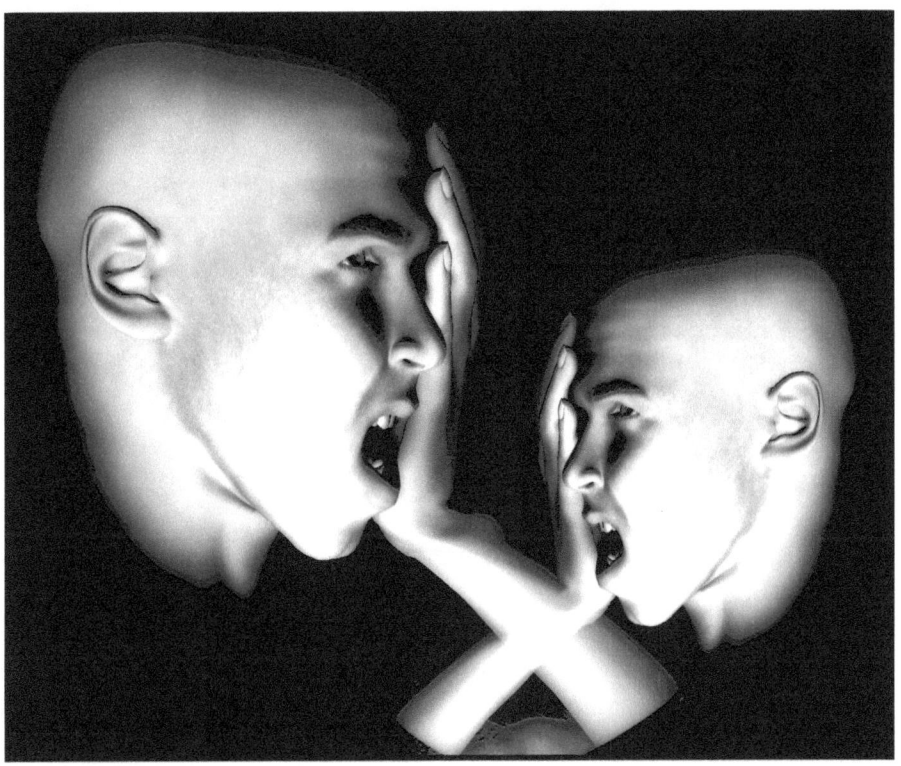

Illustration 13: Mental illness is so hard to live with. Why make it harder by eating refined sugars and poisoning your body and brain?

Trying to determine which one caused which (the sugar or the depression) is a bit like the chicken-and-the-egg discussion. But there is no question that refined sugar can cause or deepen a person's depression.

If you are a person who suffers from depression, if you have been diagnosed as bipolar, or suffer from any other psychosis, this is not something you probably enjoy hearing. Telling you to cut out sugar, our favorite comfort food, is probably not the answer you were looking for. And it is definitely not the only answer. Most likely, your illness is caused by a combination of factors that will each need to be addressed. And you should not stop consulting professional help. However, I sincerely believe that cutting out all refined sugar can help you calm the emotional swings and help you to feeling better about life. At a minimum, it can lessen the mood swings and give you a better chance at dealing with the source of the problem. Perhaps in time, you might even be able to live free from your depression which would be the ultimate goal. And when I say to cut out refined sugars, I am including foods that are processed with sugar as the preservative and foods that turn quickly into sugar in your blood like white flour and white starches.

Much of why refined sugar affects the mood is what we've already discussed in chapter four and sugar's similarities to heroin. Sugar can deepen and increase the frequency of the lows that you feel. The presence of too much sugar in the blood also boosts the serotonin levels, significantly affecting your moods. Unbalanced serotonin levels can wreak havoc on one's mental stability.

In closing, if you have been diagnosed as bipolar or suffer from any other psychological or emotional issues, I can't see anything but a benefit for you to take *The Dare* and cut out refined sugars. It certainly won't do as much damage as the drugs used to manage the depression. Take this from one who was mildly prone to depression myself in the past. Depression can be such a hard thing to come out of and you want to give yourself the best chance as possible.

***

Diabetes

"Today, sugar is a virtual staple of the American diet. In fact, for many of us, a normal day includes one or two desserts. And sugar is found not just in the dessert foods like cookies and cake, but in cereals, salad dressings, processed meats, and other foods. Add to that the regular consumption of high-sugar sodas and sugar-sweetened tea and coffee, and you can get a rate of sugar consumption that is unprecedented in human history. Not surprisingly then, our bodies are not adapted to handle the barrage of sugar we regularly face. Excessive sugar consumption can create a chronic dysfunction in sugar metabolism. For some people, this dysfunction can lead to excessive high blood sugar . . ."

Natural Relief for Anxiety by Edmund J. Bourus, PhD
Arlen Brownstein, ND and Lorna Garano

For those of you who don't already know, diabetes is a blood sugar disorder where the body struggles regulating a healthy level of blood sugar. Generally, there are two types of diabetes: type 1, which is also called early onset diabetes; and type 2 diabetes, otherwise known as late-onset diabetes.

Diabetes accounts for about 5% of the deaths in the world today and is expected to increase over 50% in the next decade. It has reached epidemic proportions in the United States. According to the Center for Disease Control (CDC)[††††††††], diabetes affects more than 25.8 million of the 300+ million Americans, or 8.3 % of the population. That is almost three times the population of New York City, the largest city in the U.S. by population! This chronic disease was the seventh leading cause of death listed on U.S. death certificates in 2006, though it is likely to be underreported since the risk of death among diabetics from other related causes is twice that of non-diabetics. Speaking of other related diseases, diabetes is also one of the top causes of heart disease, the number one killer in the U.S., as well as stroke. In 2010 alone, 1.9 million people were newly diagnosed with diabetes. Now those are some unpleasant statistics.

In terms of the causes of diabetes, the CDC tells us that lack of exercise and obesity combined account for 95% of all cases . . . 95%! Just think, if we could take care of those two areas in our life, New York City could be cured of diabetes . . . three times! When it comes to exercise, my motto is "the best type of exercise one can do is the one they do." It really doesn't matter what you do as long as you are getting your heart rate up and that you are sweating. The problem is this: People spend all this money at a nice gym; they buy the new running shoes and sporty-looking outfits but only go to the gym once a week. And once they are there, they bounce around from machine to machine, never really getting their heart rate up and never breaking more than a glisten. You'd be better off going walking outside with your significant others and saving the money that you are spending. I think that if

---

[††††††††] 2011 National Diabetes Fact Sheet (pdf) found on http://www. cdc.gov/diabetes/pubs/factsheet11.htm

you will simply dedicate yourself to being more active in all areas of your life, you will notice a difference. Take the stairs instead of the elevator, even in a hotel. Park in the farthest space from the building, forcing yourself to walk more. Go out and work in your yard more. Find a physical hobby that you like such as hiking or biking. Take the family to the park instead of sitting in front of the TV. You will have more fun together and better opportunities to develop a relationship.

When it comes to obesity, I've already briefly discussed the topic above. But isn't it interesting how all of these chronic illnesses are connected. Once you understand inflammation and how it is one of the underlying causes of our illnesses, the pieces all start fitting together. Let me recommend again Dr. Duke Johnson's book called *The Optimal Health Revolution*. I believe that is one of the best overviews of the factors that affect our health, to include diabetes, obesity, and the role of inflammation.

I had a coworker in one of my first jobs who had type 2 diabetes. She resented the condition because she had certain lifestyle choices that she did not want to let go — sweets and alcohol (which both turn into glucose in the blood). My coworker was a female, and she and her husband often would go out to eat after work, have some desert and a few drinks with friends. It was one of her favorite things to do. I knew this because she would often talk about it. But as her condition progressed, she began having more and more problems. It was not uncommon for me to hear some story about how she had been out and ended up in the hospital after a diabetic episode. She had thrown up, forgotten where she was, gotten confused and almost got in a car accident, and even passed out. I eventually moved on from that position and don't know what became of my coworker. I hope she came to accept her condition and made some changes.

The point to this story is that it is my belief that though the sensitivity to the sugars was probably a genetic predisposition, my friend could have prevented the predisposition from "playing out" in her body. It was her lifestyle that developed the condition — specifically the severity of it.

Another example of burnout as it relates to diabetes is with my own grandfather. My grandfather had type 2 diabetes as well. In fact, not only did he have it, but his five brothers and sisters had it, all of them the late-onset type. I remember sitting around watching TV with my grandfather in his wheelchair because he'd had both legs amputated due to poor blood circulation from his diabetes. They actually took the legs in stages. It all started when my grandfather had put his foot in a shoe that had a golf ball in it and he didn't even notice. He wore the shoe for a long time without feeling it. Eventually, he got an infection that ended in the first amputation — his foot. The rest progressed from there.

Looking at my grandfather's lifestyle, his diet was full of meat and potatoes, alcohol, and sugar — foods that turn to glucose in the blood. I have to wonder whether he could have prolonged his life (God-willing) if he would have managed his diet better, exercised more, and cut out the starches and refined sugars. His condition of diabetes might have taken a lot longer to progress without burning out his pancreas. Amazingly, he lived to age 79. It would have been nice to have had him until 90!

So when all of these cases of diabetes come across the examining tables of our medical professionals, what do they recommend? Insulin! Oh yes, many if not most of these doctors are telling their patients to cut down on refined sugars, but what they should be telling people is to cut out refined sugars for the rest of their lives. When you tell a person that it is OK to continue their destructive eating habits by only cutting back a little, you are shortening their lives. You don't tell a heroin addict to just cut back, do you? A person whose pancreas is overly sensitive to sugars can really live a normal life if they will just cut out the refined sugars before the pancreas is damaged beyond repair. It does not kill a person not to eat refined sugars. It does kill them to eat refined sugars on a regular basis in large amounts.

***

Cardiovascular Disease (aka Heart Disease)

"Diabetes and pre-diabetes cause inflammation and hardening of the arteries. High levels of glucose in blood, even short-term spikes after a meal, can have many undesirable effects and are a predictor of future heart disease . . . High insulin levels also increase the tendency for blood clots to form . . ."

The New Glucose Revolution by Dr. Jennie Brand-Miller, Dr. Thomas M. S. Wolever, Kaye Foster-Powell, And Dr. Stephen Colagiuri

This is quite a statement above. These authors also state that " . . . knowing your blood glucose level is just as important as knowing your cholesterol level to be able to ensure optimum heart health." Again, we are not saying that the removal of refined sugars from your diet alone will eliminate your chances of having heart disease. However, there are strong correlations between diabetes and heart disease, as there are strong correlations between obesity and diabetes . . .

Are you starting to see the connections?

The body is not that difficult to understand, when you think about how it is supposed to work as a whole. There is no diabetes germ. There is no obesity germ or a heart-disease germ. Unless there is a congenital issue, a pharmaceutically-caused issue, an environmental issue, or something of the sort, heart disease is caused by lifestyle, particularly one's level of stress, habits of activity, and diet. When you consider the amount of sugar that the average American intakes per year and the fact that over 60% of Americans are overweight, 20% excessively overweight, it is not hard to perceive the connections.

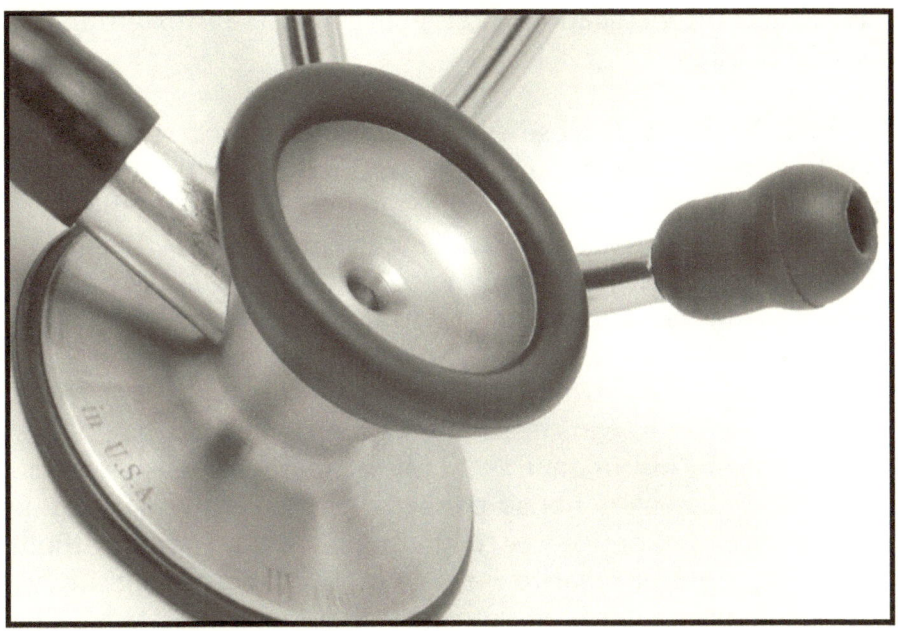

Illustration 14: Stethoscope for monitoring the heart

***

The Common Cold/Flu/Virus

Like most people, you have suffered from the occasional seasonal cold or flu. Today, it is common for people to get a flu shot during the peak flu seasons. Whenever the seasons start changing, that is when people start getting sick. This is nothing new.

But lately, I have been noticing something that seems a little off. With all of the disinfectant sprays, disinfectant soaps, disinfectant cleaners, etc., it is becoming apparent that people are beginning to believe that the reason they get sick is because of the appearance of a pathogen (germ). This explains why people will go to the doctor any time they have a "sniffly" nose or get a low-grade fever. It also explains why people rush out to the store to buy the over-the-counter medicines as soon as they feel the slight bit ill. They believe that something has gotten into the body, and they have to take the medication to get rid of it, just like an exterminator gets rid of bugs.

But I would like to propose a different thought process. I propose that the germs have been getting into the body all along. The presence of the germ was not what made you sick. Yes, the germ has to be there to be sick. But what made you sick and what makes you feel bad is that your immune system is too weak to fight off the germ that got in your body, and the germ was allowed to multiply over and over again. The fact is that germs are in every square inch of air. Throughout our day, especially if we are out in public, we breathe in germs or get germs on our food and now we have them in our mouth. Many of these germs would kill us if our bodies were not so perfectly created that our immune systems already knows how to kill and eliminate germs without us having to tell it what to do. Think about it, even right now, you could have a germ on your tongue or in your stomach that even now is being killed, and you don't even know it. Every time a germ gets through our outer defenses (skin mostly), the body sends the army to surround this germ and swallow it up. These army men are called our white blood cells. But what is even more amazing is that our bodies create antibodies after they've defeated their foe, which are puzzlelike pieces that are an exact match to the germ that they just killed. Now, when the germ enters the body, it is much quicker and easier to kill.

So how does refined sugar affect getting sick? If we get sick because our immune system is low, then anything that we can do to keep our immune system strong is good. On the other hand, anything we do that weakens our immune system increases our chances of being sick. One of the things I noticed when I cut out sugars was that I did not get sick nearly as often as before; maybe once every few years and usually nothing more than a cold. The truth is that many people get sick more often than they should because of lifestyle, diet being a big part of this. And considering that sugar is such a large part of the American diet today and that it has been proven to lower the immune system, I would think twice about having that energy drink with sugar while you are fighting off a cold or taking that cold medicine made with sugar.

Refined sugar robs the body of essential vitamins and minerals that are needed by the body to fight off disease. Sugar is also an acid and therefore creates a more germ-friendly environment, germs thriving in a more acidic atmosphere. I'm not saying don't take medication. There are many wonderful medicines that help save lives and make people's lives better. All I'm saying is to help your body be healthy; don't hinder it by eating or drinking sugar.

For most people these days, life is getting busier and busier. Time is not a luxury that many have. And having to take time off of work for being sick is something you would rather not have to do. I would recommend, especially if you are prone to seasonal colds or the flu, take *The Dare* and cut out the refined sugars. Try doing it during the times that you normally get sick and see if you get better faster or get less sick. I would start it about a month before the sick season and then just continue on. See what a difference it will make!

***

Headaches

> *"When the blood sugar falls too low or too rapidly, a patient experiences symptoms such as lightheadedness, weakness, headache, sweating, and change in level of consciousness if the condition is severe enough."*[††††††††]

The National Headache Foundation

There can be many reasons why people get headaches, and if you suffer from regular headaches, you should look into all possible factors. There are great resources out there that can help you in that search. As it applies to sugar, headaches can be greatly affected by a high sugar consumption. Depending on the person, this could be partly due to the drastic fluctuations in blood sugar.

[††††††††] http://www.headaches.org/education/Headache_Topic_Sheets/Hypoglycemia

If you've just flooded your body with a large dose of sugar and the blood sugar has dropped from the large amounts of insulin to make the body absorb the sugar, you go into a deep low with little energy to do what you need to. The body can go into a panic mode when this happens and produce adrenalin to keep up your energy. Adrenaline can cause headaches. Talk about putting your body through a roller-coaster ride!

The headaches can be more of a secondary result as well. When I was a teenager, I used to get mild headaches. They were manageable by taking over-the-counter medication. But by the time I was getting out of college, the headaches continued to get worse. In my late twenties, they were so bad that I would have to leave work early or miss out on family outings to stay home and sleep it off. My headaches would be so bad that they would keep me up all night, tossing and turning. I could never get comfortable. I would hit my head with books and try anything to get the pain to stop. I couldn't even open my eyes because the light made it worse. I remember telling my wife once that if I had a drill, I would drill into my head if I knew it would relieve the pain. (Please don't ever try that. It won't work.)

I didn't have headaches all the time, and I just learned to live with them. But it wasn't until I was forced to cut out refined sugars, white flour, and white starches that my headaches went away. One of the reasons I believe this happened is that I was suffering from a magnesium deficiency. Magnesium is something that you have to get from eating as it is not created by the body. Oftentimes it is combined with calcium in a vitamin pill as the two are essential together for proper absorption. During the years of my headaches, I was eating and drinking a lot of sugary, starchy, and processed foods. I was also taking in a lot of caffeine in sodas and coffee. Caffeine is known to sap the body of magnesium, along with sugar. I was a particularly high-strung person at the time and stress also decreases magnesium in the body.

Once I cut out the refined sugars, my migraines slowly went away. Sugar was not the only thing I cut out, though. I also cut out coffee and began supplementing the magnesium. So it is difficult to say which change made the most difference. Interestingly, I was still drinking tea, so I was still getting caffeine. But either way, the headaches went away. Today, when I start feeling the beginning of a headache, I make sure I take my supplements; and of course I make sure that I am not eating any sugar to make sure all factors are eliminated.

One thing I want to reiterate, as I mentioned in chapter two, I didn't just accept my headaches. I went on a journey to figure out how to rid myself of them. And since there are so many things in the body that affect each other, it was no surprise to me that healing one issue inadvertently cured another.

If you are suffering from headaches, after consulting your doctor, you might want to try taking *The Dare* and to see if it helps. I can't fully say that cutting out the refined sugar by itself will rid you of the headaches. But it is a good start. And by combining it with other items like supplementing, a good chiropractor, etc., I believe it would make a big difference. It can't hurt you to try; and isn't it better to try and fail than it is to have never tried and to have no hope? I believe so.

Our Own Son's Story

When we adopted our son, he was five and a half years old and diagnosed with attention deficit disorder and hyperactivity, a common diagnosis among foster children. He had been prescribed Ritalin and had already had his dosage increased twice in the prior year per teacher, foster mother, doctor agreement.

In school, he struggled to pay attention, threw rocks on the playground, and had to be seated by himself to keep from bothering his peers, despite repeated negative consequences. His academic progress was slow to the point of needing to be retained in kindergarten. His foster mother described similar behaviors at home including inability to focus on homework and high levels of hyperactivity.

Upon our visit to his school, we noticed that part of his daily schedule included eating ice cream instead of a healthy snack. We also visited his foster home. As all of the kids sat around sipping sodas and eating popsicles, we watched our son bounce from activity to activity, unable to maintain focus for more than a few minutes. For dinner, they ate boxed macaroni and cheese along with dessert despite already having had popsicles after school.

I'm not saying you should do this, but when he came to live with us, we did two things: We weaned him off his medication, and we set in place the no-sugar policy. Initially, he was very resistant without sugar but gradually became accustomed to it (our kids are living proof that a child who was thought to be "picky," will eat what you put in front of them if there is no other option and usually begin to enjoy it!). As he finished the school year, he showed no signs of the previous behavioral issues. Other than being a bit too talkative, the teacher reported that he was able to focus and was a hard worker.

We know the root of these issues were more emotional in nature, but it certainly hindered our son from being able to feel good and to focus. Giving him candy was like pouring gasoline on a fire. Today, at age seven, he is able to focus so well that he will sit reading for an hour at a time and reads a year above grade level.

Tony Gonzalez

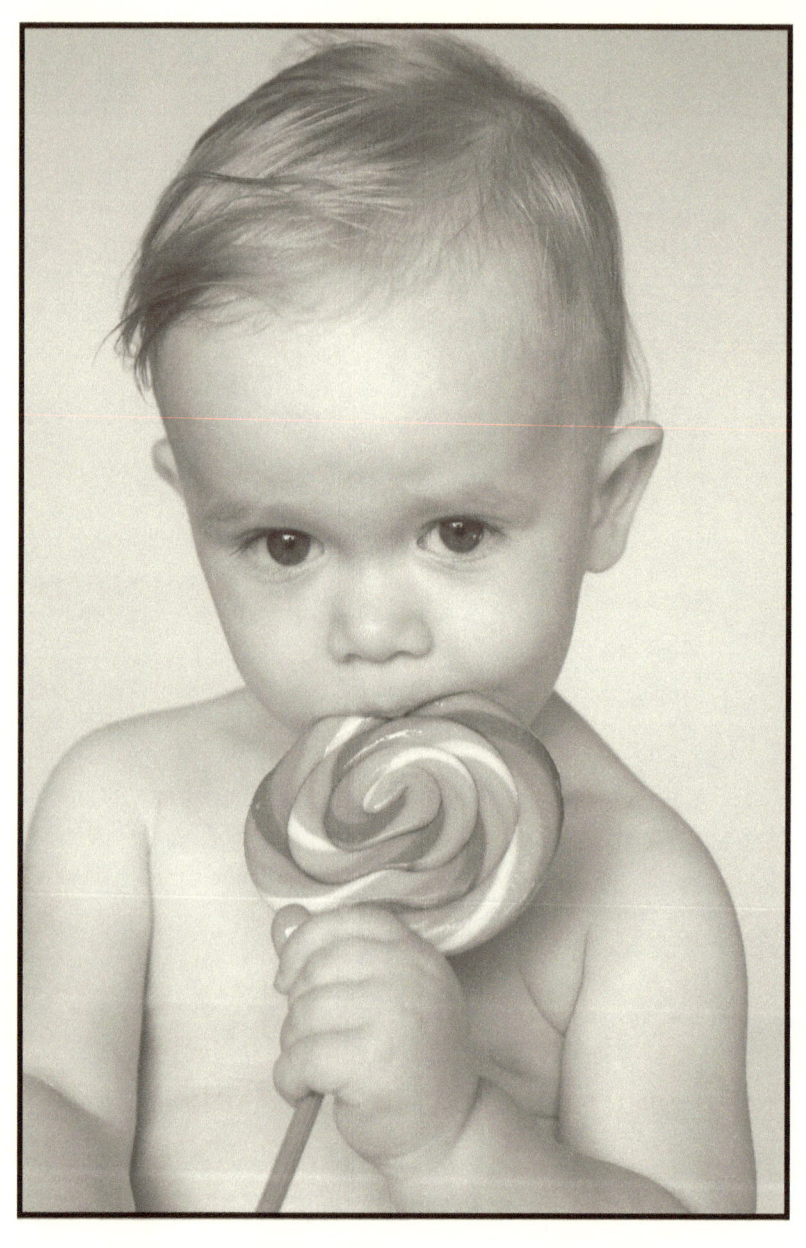

Illustration 15: Have you ever known a child to
turn down a lollipop? Not likely.

Chapter 7: Children and Sugar

" . . . the food (that we usually find at a classroom birthday party, school meeting, etc.) is a good example of what parents unknowingly do to make kids struggle in school. Most children start the day with muffins, donuts, Pop-tarts, bagels, cinnamon rolls, and sugary cereals. They get virtually no protein in the morning. No wonder teachers complain that half the kids can't concentrate. In order for children or adults to focus, they need to have nutritious food that enhances energy concentration. Especially for people with ADD, the solution is a higher protein, lower carbohydrate diet."

Healing ADD—
The Breakthrough Program that Allows You to See and Heal the Six Types
of ADD by Daniel G. Amen, MD pp. 223-224

This topic was the original reason why this book was written. It was originally intended to be a simple twenty – to thirty-page pamphlet. I wanted something that I could give people to help explain why my wife and I didn't let our children eat the birthday cake at their cousin's birthday party, the Halloween candy after trick-or-treating, or the cookies at Christmas. As you can see, it has turned into more than just a pamphlet. But when I got to writing this chapter, I thought that my wife, Katie, would be better suited for this, having been a teacher for fourteen years on top of being a parent for over thirteen years. Like me, Katie is passionate about children and giving them the best start possible at living a full and meaningful life. Having worked within the foster care systems in New Mexico and Georgia, as well as having adopted our own four children out of foster care, I believe Katie has a lot of credibility and a unique perspective when dealing with children. So here is my wife's take on this . . .

When our now fourteen-year-old was around three, Tony and I had an "ah-ha" moment. I remember clearly, we were out on a late lunch date with our extended family and our daughter had a hotdog with white bun, fries, a sugary dessert, and lemonade. What Tony and I noticed on that day was how drastically our daughter changed from a calm, polite child into a whirlwind.

After she ate her food, she became spastic and was laughing maniacally. When told to calm down, she would just hop up and down next to our table in a frenzy of activity. To confuse us even more, forty-five minutes later she was a limp noodle, grouchy and fussy over every little thing. This was many hours before bedtime, and she had taken a good nap that day. At the time, we had no idea what was going on. All we knew was that our child became a different person after eating some foods, but we weren't sure which ones. All we had pieced together at the time was that it seemed to have something to do with what she ate.

To continue on with the story, the next morning our daughter was nauseous and extremely shaky, having only eaten a snack for dinner the night before. We decided to go to the doctor to test her for diabetes. The doctor informed us that our daughter was hypoglycemic as well as allergic to specific foods. He told us to cut out all dairy and sugars, including juice. He told us that her body did not tolerate too many simple sugars. We followed his directions, and it has made a huge difference in our daughter's behavior and overall health. From then on, her moods and energy levels stayed relatively consistent.

**

IT STARTS AT HOME

As a parent and teacher, one of the things I want to reiterate here is how important a good diet is to the wellbeing of our children, both physically and mentally. As Tony mentioned at the beginning of this book, what we eat really does affect our health. What I find so frustrating is how often I see a child with attention problems, hyperactivity issues, or even health issues eating "foods"§§§§§§§§ that are either causing the problem or making the problem much worse than it has to be. It all starts at home. We as a nation need to start looking at what we feed our children and consider the

---

§§§§§§§§ I put "food" in quotes because today we call anything that we put into our mouths food. In reality, only the stuff that is good for us should be called food.

long term affects. According to the Center for Disease Control, the number of obese children and adolescents has almost tripled since 1980, going from around 6% of all children to 17%. Seventeen percent is 12.5 million children and adolescents ranging in age from two to nineteen![¶¶¶¶¶¶¶¶] And obesity is just one issue dealing with the diets of our children.

Tony has already discussed some of the physical effects of obesity, but until recently most of these issues were happening to adults. Today, however, we are seeing them in children. And I don't know about you, but to see high blood pressure or type 2 diabetes in a five-year-old just seems wrong to me, especially when the child can barely run because they are overweight. When we start seeing health issues that are usually adult issues coming up in our children, it should make us step back and rethink whether we are holding up our part of the parenting. If we truly love our children, we would give them healthy habits to carry into adulthood. And if our own habits are not healthy, we should be willing to change for the sake of our children. If your child is overweight and has heartburn, acid reflux, sleep apnea, it is time to make a change. I'm not saying this to be judgmental; I'm saying it because I care about children and their families and want to see them happy and healthy.

Everywhere you turn, foods that are full of simple carbohydrates and refined sugars are being pushed on our children; and we wonder why our children are suffering from chronic diseases. It all starts in the morning. Sugary cereals, prepackaged lunches, purple catsup, fruitlike rolls—these are all common "foods" found in the common American child's breakfast diet today. Tarts with "fruity" fillings are a favorite breakfast for many. It used to be my favorite. Have you ever looked at the ingredients, though? You will find that white flour and sugar are the two main ingredients, along with some other things that you can't even pronounce. Just take a look at the ingredients on the pre-made or ready-made muffins . . . sugar. And it is not much better with a "healthy" cereal! Look at the ingredients on the box and you

---

¶¶¶¶¶¶¶¶ http://www.cdc.gov/obesity/childhood/data.htm

will still see sugar as the main ingredient. In fact, it is very hard to find any cereal that does not use sugar. It might be organic, unbleached sugar, and there might be other great ingredients, but there is sugar nonetheless. And what about oatmeal, oatmeal is healthy, right? But how many people do you know who eat oatmeal without sugar? (Check out our sugar-free oatmeal recipe at the end of this book!)

As parents, we say we want our kids to succeed in school, but yet we provide them with foods that are totally devoid of nutrition, foods that run their poor little bodies through a blood sugar rollercoaster and that turn them into an unfocused and unmotivated child. That is how we are sending our kids to school every day.

SCHOOL FOOD

I have had many people scoff when I said children's behaviors changed after having sugar. If you ever come to an elementary school lunchroom, the first thing you will notice is that the noise level is almost that of a rock concert! If you observe the food more closely, you will notice the large quantities of sugars and other simple carbohydrates in the lunch boxes and school lunches. As a teacher who has probably seen thousands of children before and after lunch, I can honestly say that children's behavior can and does change due to what they eat.

Looking at the lunches brought from home, I've seen lunch boxes carrying food items that more resemble vending machine snacks than good, nutritious food; breakfast tarts or a sugary cereal for the main entrée; cookies and a fake fruit substance for their side. And to wash it all down, they have "fruit" punch, low on the fruit and high on the sugar. Oftentimes, they have a white bread sandwich with peanut butter and jelly, both with added sugar. Mom and dad might try to get something healthy into the lunchbox, so they toss in a fruit cup; but the fruit is packaged in light syrup (sugar). And who doesn't love the fruit roll or fruit gummies, which are essentially candy that we like to pretend are somewhat related to a fruit.

But what about all of those children who eat the school lunches? Well, the typical school lunch consists of one main course and two side dishes. The children could choose the one main dish from four different options, generally having some sort of meat and bread (typically white bread). At the last school where I taught, they had five or six different side dishes to choose from. There is one canned vegetable choice and several canned fruit choices in light syrup (sugar, also works as a preservative). On many occasions, the fruit option would include a fruit-flavored popsicle, fries, tater tots, and sometimes a cookie. Of course, the only drink offered is milk because of the lack of calcium in the average American diet. But it is not just plain milk, though, that is offered. There are many choices here as well. Strawberry milk, chocolate milk, ice milk, and vanilla milk—all with a sugar content that is enough to make any child hyper. On top of that, ice cream is a regular tool for schools to raise money as a fundraiser and to enforce behavioral discipline in schools. How many children do you know that turn down ice cream when given the opportunity?

After coming into the lunchroom and noticing the food, you might then turn to the children's behavior. On most days, we would leave the classroom orderly and calm. The children would enter the lunchroom as quietly as kindergarteners can, sit down, and begin to eat. As the minutes ticked by, the kids begin to get more and more active. Louder and louder they would get. A typical lunchtime was only thirty minutes. But once their time was over, getting these same children who were attentive and calm thirty minutes ago to clean up their trash and take their tray was an exercise in patience. Just getting their attention was difficult.

Once their trays have hopefully made it to the trash can without spilling, the children are then instructed to walk in a line, something they could do relatively well before lunch. After lunch, however, the children tend to jostle around, pick on each other, and incite chaos! Many of the kids begin to run into rooms that they have been told every day since they started kindergarten not to run into. Inevitably, someone slips and falls and someone else starts a pushing fight so they can be first in line to the water fountain or rest room. Of course, just standing in line is almost out of the question! It's as if the quiet, calm children that were dropped off for lunch have been replaced with Mexican jumping beans!

As we make our way down the hall, the children are putting their lunchboxes on their heads, jumping instead of walking, and generally having trouble controlling themselves. Once they are in the room, many have difficulty sitting and concentrating. In less than an hour, these hyper kids begin to crash. I've heard many teachers say that "once lunch is over, the kids are useless for the rest of the day. The most and best learning takes place before lunch." I would argue that the reason this happens is due to what they have eaten. When you are watching, it is pretty easy to notice. The children whose parents send in healthy lunches generally leave the lunchroom the same way they came in and are able to focus and work when returning to the class setting. I'm not saying that kindergarteners don't ever put their lunch box on their head or get into a pushing fight and I'm not saying that they only do this because they ate sugar. I am saying that the number of children who appear visibly different after lunch compared to before is obvious to those watching.

**

But what about our after-school activities, when we run off to sports, dance, and music lessons. We're juggling five different things before bedtime, so we run through the closest fast food place, pay too much for fake food, and eat it on the run. Can you say heartburn? At the ballpark, the kids drink a sugar-filled sports drink that is actually two servings in one so it has twice the sugar mentioned on the label. Then we get to go home and attempt to concentrate on homework? How many of us are familiar with this struggle?

As a teacher and parent, I would recommend any family to take The Dare. We originally did it as a family to support my husband who was having the health issues that you read about. But in the end, I realized that I felt better by having taken The Dare.

Originally, it was not easy. We essentially had to redefine our favorite recipes for holidays, birthdays, and everyday meals. But the health that we have all enjoyed has made it well worth the challenge of changing. Our children, my husband, and I rarely ever get sick, and when we do, it only lasts a few days.

So take *The Dare*. Instead of thinking of it as a punishment, think of it as a fun challenge to come up with foods that are fun but don't have refined sugar. You will find that there are plenty of wonderful foods that taste great and are much healthier than refined sweeteners. Even if only one family changes their lifestyle and creates the proper dietary habits for their kids, this book and the efforts that have been made to produce it will have been more than worth it!

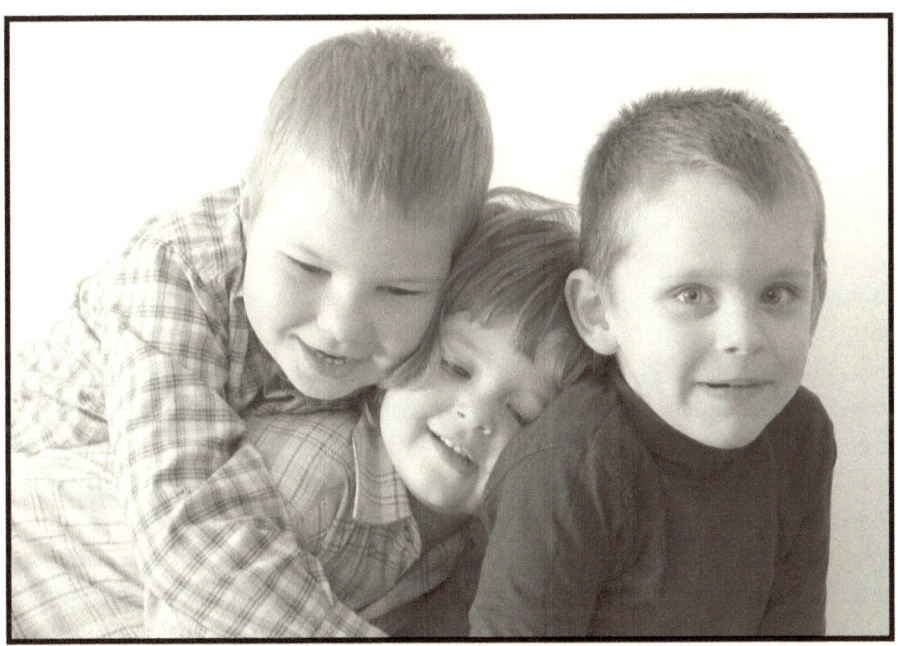

Illustration 16: Boys by themselves have a lot of energy,
but when you add sugar to the mix, it becomes explosive,
to use my wife's description.

**

HYPERACTIVITY AND ADD

Let's discuss a real hot-topic: hyperactivity and ADD. This is one of those issues that teachers love to complain about but hate to hear about. The range of opinions on the topic is wide and the emotions strong. Many will say that I'm oversimplifying the problem in what I am about to say. I'm aware that there can be numerous factors that can cause the same symptoms as ADD/ ADHD (food allergies such as gluten, emotional situations, too much screen time). But I've taught many children, including my own son, who were diagnosed ADD or ADHD. Most were on medication by the time they got to first grade. And most ate, what in preventative health circles has been dubbed, a SAD diet or "standard American diet." This includes the fast food, the simple carbs, and of course the sugary foods. Did you know the two most consumed vegetables in the U.S.? Tomatoes and potatoes in the form of catsup and french fries (sugars and starches)!

While I know there are times when medication is necessary and life-saving, when it comes to our children, I have to wonder if we are not misdiagnosing or overmedicating our children when the solution could be much simpler and healthier. Dr. Kim John Payne, MEd, who wrote the book *Simplicity Parenting*, states: "We've fully embraced the pharmacological approach to behavioral issues in America; there are now more than 7 million children taking Ritalin. No other country prescribes psychoactive medications to children the way we do; Americans consume 80% of the world's Ritalin."[*] That's pretty staggering! One of my teacher friends went to a school in Tanzania for two weeks to teach some continuing education classes for their staff. While there, she noticed classrooms of approximately forty children as young as kindergarten sitting politely, focused on the task at hand. When they went out to play or eat, they quickly came back to class and refocused. This was consistent through the school during her

---

[*] *Simplicity Parenting*, by Dr. Kim John Payne, MEd, Ballantine Books. ©2009.

whole visit. Her comment when she came back was, "There is no ADD in Africa." I'm sure there are other factors involved, but it is interesting to note that there is far less processed food or sugar readily available!

Over the years, I've been suggesting to parents that they try different dietary restrictions for their child who was struggling with focus or hyperactivity. I included cutting sugar entirely from their diet. Frequently, however, parents would look at me as if I were crazy, mostly (I believe) because they couldn't see themselves living without sugar. Others would flatly say, "Oh, we tried that and it didn't really help." Typically, when I hear someone say this, they either tried cutting out sugar for a few days and quit because they didn't see immediate results *or* they never really tried and discount it because it is not something they wanted to do in the first place. I find it interesting how there is so much evidence of the damage refined sugar can do to the body, yet there are so many parents who are not willing to protect their kids from the effects because they might have to cut sugar out as well from their own diet.

**

CONCLUSION

I've watched parents give their children junk food and candy, then claim their kids won't eat healthy food. While their children's taste buds prefer the sugar, their growing bodies and developing brains prefer good nutrition. I'd actually go so far as to say that their bodies and brains are not going to develop properly without this good nutrition! The scary part is that we as parents ingrain the future habits of our children. In terms of health and nutrition, we create these habits as well, both good and bad. Our children have no control in the matter until they are old enough to monitor their own habits. By then, the bad habits have already been developed and are hard to change. Once bad habits are created, it takes a lot of effort to change them, and most people simply don't have enough desire.

All we have to do is look around and we can find people struggling with their children. Their children won't listen. Their children are manipulative and play emotional games to get what they want. Their children are disobedient and disrespectful. Part of the problem is that we have a nation that practices permissive parenting, letting the children dictate what is best. But I really believe that part of the problem is simply that we are drugging our kids with sugar and then drugging them again because they are not focused. Let's just go back to the days before ADD and medication and look at what children ate. If we teach our children good foundational habits of nutrition, and they see us following those habits as well, they are much more likely to enter adulthood as healthy eaters!

Again, if you and your family regularly eat sugar, if you have sodas, snack cakes, brownies, sugary cereals, and sports energy drinks in your house, it is time to break the family free from the sugar bondage. Make it a fun challenge instead of a dreaded diet. Experiment together and come up with foods that are fun and tasty but which don't have refined sugar. Begin changing what I call your "food repertoire." Find new recipes that you like but that are healthier. Take *The Dare* as a family. You will be thankful you did!

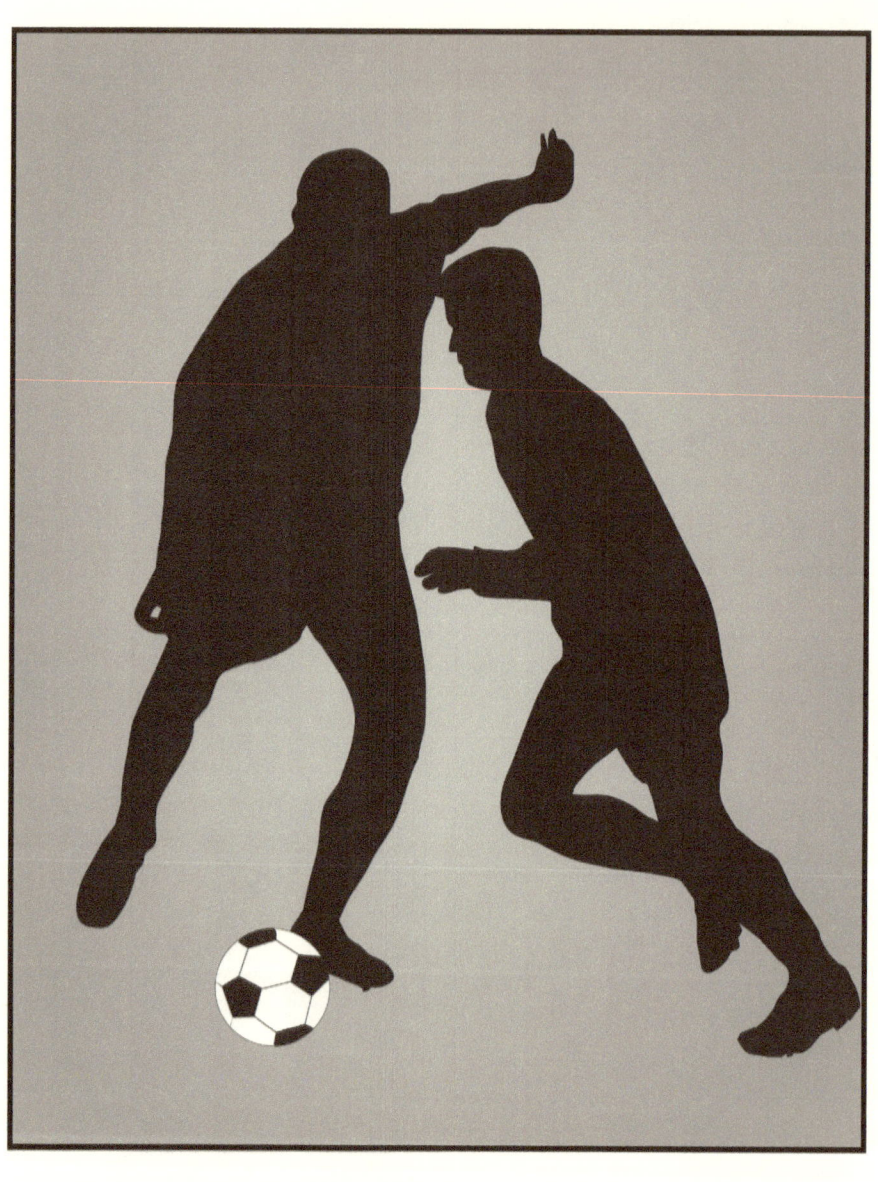

Illustration 17: Refined sugar may improve the performance
of these players, but what are the long term effects?

Chapter 8: Athletics and Sugar

Does Sugar Give You Energy?

When I was young, I used to play sports. I played soccer and baseball. I was only missing two key components or I could have gone far: talent and ability. If it wasn't for the lack of those two things, I might have made it to the professional level. In all seriousness, out of all of the sports I played, I played soccer the longest. I remember at halftime, we would have some sort of a snack that was brought in by one of the parents. The purpose of the snack was to help keep up our energy for the second half of the game. I always hoped for the parents who brought orange slices. When you are running non-stop, orange slices are so refreshing.

But thinking back, there were always two main groups of parents who brought snacks: those who brought fruit and those that brought sugar. The ones from the fruit camp brought oranges, bananas, apples, and grapes accompanied by water. The ones in the sugar camp brought candy bars with juice or sports drinks. I always enjoyed the candy bars; who wouldn't? But when you were tired from running and sweating, nothing felt as refreshing as the fruit.

But this brings up a good question about sugar and energy. Does sugar give us energy? And furthermore, as it relates to sports, does sugar increase performance? I regularly hear people mention that they are dragging in energy and use eating candy as the solution. There are lots of coaches who prescribe candy bars at halftime or before the game to "fill up" with energy. Athletes, such as marathon runners and bikers are constantly eating sugar bars and sugary drinks for "quick energy" while on their long bike rides, swims, or runs. So according to them, sugar does give you energy. And we all know that candy is known to make a child hyper. Many of us have felt what it is like to have a sugar-high after taking the kids trick-or-treating or going to a fair and eating cotton candy. So from our own personal experience I think most people would agree that, at a minimum, sugar does initially make a person feel more energetic. Of course, this is until the blood sugar decreases again. But when it comes to athletic performance, does sugar boost our performance . . . or do we just think it does?

Originally, I wanted to provide a more clear-cut answer about this question; I love issues that are black and white. So I put together a test. I have a chiropractor friend who has a machine that can measure physical strength. He uses it to test the strength of muscles before and after adjustments. I asked my friend if I could use this machine to measure refined sugar's effect on muscle strength. After gaining his approval, I had thirteen people (test subjects) meet me at the office one morning. To make sure they were not already under the influence of sugar, I had them abstain from eating or drinking anything the day of the test. That at least gave me eight or more hours without sugar. I performed three tests on each of the thirteen participants: leg lift, arm lift, and shoulder lift. To prevent any influence on each other, I had each person perform the tests separately.

To work the machine the person presses as hard as they can on a pad set up in a certain position and holds that position for ten seconds. The machine then measures and calculates the maximum force that is applied during that time. One at a time I had each participant come into the room, get on the machine, and perform the tests. Then I gave each person one packet of raw, granulated cane sugar. I had them all put the sugar under their tongue and let it dissolve. Most of them winced, saying it was a lot of sugar, which is interesting because they put one or two of these in a cup of coffee. I gave them one minute after eating the sugar and then ran the tests again.

My hypothesis was that, though the person might have a sense of heightened awareness and energy mentally, that the muscle strength would actually decrease rapidly as the body had to deal with the sudden surge of blood sugar. Unfortunately, the results were not as clear-cut as I originally thought. There was no trend whatsoever that would indicate any real finding. My scientific experiment was a flop. However, performing the study did help clear up my own thoughts on the subject. I started doing research after my experiment and found some very interesting information as you will see below.

The best way to answer the question "does sugar gives you energy" is to look at what people mean by "energy." When someone says that sugar gave them energy, they can mean one of two things or, most likely, both combined. First, they might mean that it gave them improved physical ability or strength. This is the ability to jump higher, lift more weights, or run longer distances. The other possible meaning of energy is that sugar gave them mental awareness. This mental awareness is less of a physical ability and more of a state or condition of alertness or excitement. It is feeling more awake or clear-headed.

So to summarize, a person might be saying that they *are* energetic (have more energy/power) and the other person might mean that they *feel* energetic (feeling more aware). The hard part is deciphering which one it is. Also, to make things more confusing, when a person feels more energetic, they generally are more energetic. So differentiating between the two is almost impossible. There have been very interesting studies about the power of belief. Claude Bristol Myer's book, *The Power of Belief* mentions many of these studies. I remember reading about one where a person was told they were going to hold a hot iron bar on the person's hand but really held a room temperature bar on the person's hand. The amazing part is that the person developed red and blistered skin where they were touched. It was their belief that caused their body to react. Many of you might have heard of a self-fulfilling prophecy. This is when you cause something to happen simply because you believe it to be that way. For instance, if you believe you are bad at math, you subconsciously do things that verify to yourself that you are bad at math, like delay studying until the last minute because you think you are bad at it and don't enjoy it. You also don't ask questions when you don't understand things and stay out of study groups because you might get embarrassed. So in the end, because of your bad study habits that you acquired because of your belief system, you are bad at math.

When it comes to energy, when we feel like we have energy, generally we do. Whether it is the sugar that provides the energy or other chemicals in the body, such as adrenaline, it is really hard to tell. And like I already mentioned, we can all agree that sugar does, at a minimum, make us feel energetic and probably does make us more physically energetic while our blood sugar levels are up.

But what about the long-term effects? I've already talked about these effects with our society as a whole as well as discussing children and sugar. When it comes to athletes, because all bodies function the same overall, the effects of sugar are the same as well. There are, however, two differences which I believe help athletes stay healthy even though they are eating this poisonous sweet stuff. The first is that athletes sweat more than the average person. Years ago, a person would sweat more because they were working outdoors as a farmer or in a blacksmith or carpenters shop. They also didn't have artificial air, otherwise known as air-conditioning. Today, we go from our air-conditioned home to our air-conditioned car to our air—conditioned office. Rarely do we get out and sweat. Sweating helps remove the toxins in the body. When we take painkillers, eat foods with preservative and numerous other ingredients that are not commonly found in nature, or inhale the bug spray that you squirt around the house, toxins get into your body. The liver and kidneys do a great job filtering out your blood, but the toxins have to go somewhere. Oftentimes, they are stored in the fat of the body. This is one reason why a person who is fasting can feel so bad at first because the toxins in the fat of their body is releasing toxins as the fat is being burned. But these toxins can be released from the body through sweating. Sweating has been known to be healthy for centuries and is a wonderful cleansing tool.

The other difference in athletes is the more obvious: they burn more calories. Considering that we are a society with 60% of our population overweight, burning calories keeps the body weight down and helps prevent many of the issues associated with being overweight such as heart disease and cancer.

But in researching this topic of athletes and sugar, I was shocked to find out how little the correlation is even considered. There are many athletes who are "living with diabetes." In fact, there are a lot of articles about how these athletes are coping with this "disease" and still being able to compete. I think it is a great show of courage and persistence. In fact, living in Atlanta, I read about how Dominique Wilkins, the fifteen-year Hawks basketball veteran, has now been diagnosed with type 2 diabetes. I'm not trying to make light of his diagnosis, but I have to wonder could have been prevented with proper diet. I wonder how many energy drinks packed full of sugar Dominique has drunk in his lifetime. I can only speculate, not knowing Dominique, but I wonder if he keeps a diet without any refined sugars or simple carbohydrates and balanced with the proper amounts of complex carbohydrates (whole grains), proteins, fats, vitamins, and minerals. My guess is that he does not have this type of diet, and that if he did, then he wouldn't have what the doctors are calling diabetes anymore. Again, I could not say for sure as his genetics play a definite factor. He could also have other issues playing a part. But having seen it in others and having experienced it myself, his diet is more than likely playing a large factor. Even with the genetic predisposition, removal of the substance that is giving you the problem can relieve you of the problem. A person does not die without refined sugar. There are plenty of good foods to eat without refined sugars. You just have to want to be healthy enough.

So what can an athlete do for energy? For this, I think we should look at what one athlete does. Steve Nash, the two-time NBA MVP, says that he tries to stay away from foods high in refined sugars and that he gets his energy from having eaten the proper foods a week in advance.[††††††††] As an athlete, your body does need energy; but the healthiest way to do this is through a steady diet of complex carbohydrates not simple carbohydrates, fruits not candy, water not sugary drinks.

[††††††††] http://www.mensjournal.com/living-sugar-free. This is from an article written by Steve Nash that originally appeared in *Men's Journal*, Dec/Jan 2009 issue.

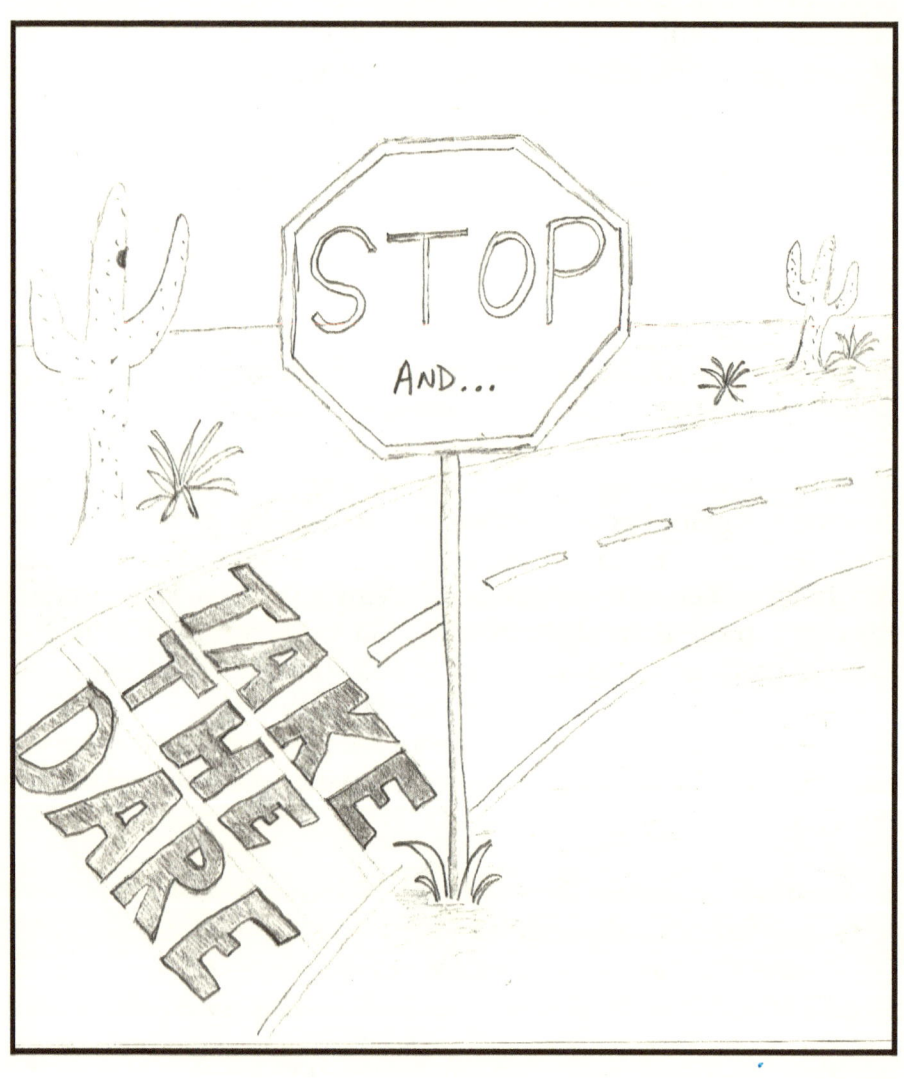

Illustration 18: Can you walk away from your
poisonous passion? Take *The Dare* and see.

Chapter 9: Wrap-up and Next Steps

OK, so you've learned what refined sugar is and what it does to our bodies. Now is the time to make the decision that will change your life by cutting out sugar. It generally is not a decision that is easy to keep, especially when you are tired and hungry; but it is certainly worthwhile.

For those of you who are ready to start, the first thing I would do is finish reading this book, including chapter ten entitled *The Dare*. Also, be sure to review the appendices as we have put together a shopping list and a one-week meal plan. Then I would go ahead and get started. Again, this is a thirty-day challenge to get you feeling the difference. It will not be easy the first week, temptations coming from everywhere. But stick to it and reap the rewards of feeling good. After all, it's only thirty days. If you can't handle thirty days, then just commit to a week at a time. That makes it a lot easier to swallow. If nothing else, this is great practice in developing and growing your self-discipline. As Plato put it so long ago, "The first and best victory is to conquer self."

After taking *The Dare* and going a month without refined sugars, if you can keep it going, great! If you are like the rest of us, you will feel the pull back to your old foods. That's the addiction talking. If you can go for another week, do it. If you can go for a few months, great! Most experts say that if you can live a sugar-free lifestyle for a year, you can break yourself of the sugar addiction, and you won't have the cravings anymore. For me, it happened before a full year. But I think my physical addiction was broken quite a while before my mental addiction. I'll talk more about that in a minute.

OK, so what do you do? Well, after you've done *The Dare*, there are a few things that would help you greatly in your journey to a healthier you. And, being the teacher that I am, I came up with an acronym to make it easy:

S – U – G – A – R

Study – Study more about this topic. Don't just take my word for it; read up on it yourself. Knowledge is power. Test it. Prove it right or wrong yourself. That is the only way you will know whether it is true or not. And let's face it, if it is true, it means all the difference in the world. After all, you only get this one time to live. Why not feel good while you are living it?

Understand – Understand that living a sugar-free lifestyle is not a diet. This is not some temporary thing you do. It is a decision to cut it out of your life. There are really two addictions that you have to break: your physical addiction and your mental addiction. The physical one, I believe, only lasts a little while, depending on whether you quit "cold turkey" or slowly cut sugar out a little bit at a time. When you've broken the physical addiction, you no longer crave the sweet concoction. Other foods start tasting better to you. Your taste buds start coming back to life. And your body starts being able to function normally. You might notice that you can handle stressful situations better. You will probably have more energy. I don't know everything that you will notice, but I do believe that you will notice significant differences.

The other addiction to break is the mental one. This is the one that took me much longer to break. This is the thought process that you are missing out if you don't partake of those wonderful doughnuts, or the triple chocolate chunk birthday cake, or the chocolate chip cookies, etc. Believe it or not, you will get to the point where you really don't crave those things; but it takes the decision that your health is more important to you than the temporary fix.

I remember while I was breaking my addiction, I would get mad at other people if they would eat sugary things around me, as if they were somehow responsible for the decision I was making. I remember in particular one Thanksgiving Day. We were all finished eating and out came the desserts. I did well not eating the candied yams nor any of the starchy things on the table. But boy, when the pecan pie, pumpkin pie, brownies, and cookies came out, I just really had a hard time. I cracked. I was grumpy and snapping at my wife over silly things. I ended up eating some of the pie and cookies out of despair. It was like I couldn't control myself. Well, because of the candida issue that I had at the time, I had a flare-up the next day and really felt bad. I was itchy and vomited in the morning. It was then that I decided that it was not worth it. I decided that I would rather be healthy and feel good than to have a temporary "feel good" session. I mean really, was it that good? When I really think about it, it wasn't. It tasted good, but you know, there are a lot of other good-tasting foods that are good for me as well. I was mentally controlled. So I made the switch and have not regretted it since.

Does that mean that I never have something with sugar in it? No. Today, I eat things with sugar in it here and there. But I don't have a romantic affair with sugar. I don't crave it, and I don't think I'm missing out when I don't have it. I believe for a time, a person needs to cut it out completely until he sells himself on the fact that he doesn't need it anymore. Once the physical and mental addictions have broken, if you have a cookie every once in a while, it won't kill you. But I warn you, if you pay attention, you'll notice that it makes you feel bad. You'll also notice that a craving will begin to creep in for another one. You have to stick to the decision, health over temporary pleasure.

Gather—Gather around yourself others who are also cutting sugar out of their diet. One of the surest ways I know of going back on one's decision to live a sugar-free lifestyle is to be around people who don't respect your decision, and worse, keep trying to get you to quit. Unfortunately, many of these people might be your family members, so you can't just get rid of them. But you can get around more people with the same desires.

Arm yourself—Arm yourself for those times that you would be tempted to join in to the sugar feast. Birthday parties, cookouts, game days, Christmas parties, Halloween parties, Valentine's Day parties, etc.—all of these have sugary items that are associated with them. And every get-together is generally going to have the same stuff. Potato chips, corn chips, M&Ms, Skittles, brownies, cookies, cake, sodas, "fruit" punch . . . and the list goes on. You have a decision to make. One choice is to go, get hungry, and dive into the sugary feast. *Or* you could plan ahead and bring something that you would eat. You could also eat before you go to the party so you won't get hungry. I know that once I get hungry, my reason goes out the window. So arm yourself and prepare!

Remove temptation—Remove the cookies, candies, brownie mixes, cake mixes, etc., from your house and remove the temptation. As this is a lifestyle change, you are now going to have to create new "favorite recipes." You can't keep the old favorites and still live a sugar-free lifestyle. I would even recommend throwing out the old cookbook and replacing it with a new, healthier one. This takes a while to get used to. There is a lot of trial and error in finding out what you like. Throughout my switchover, I discovered that I really like sugar-free granola with almond milk and a dash of stevia. I think it is better than the sugary cereals with milk I used to eat. I also love to take plain yogurt, which has sugar from the lactose, but no refined sugar, and I love to put strawberries or other fruits with a little stevia to have a really tasty treat. It is very sweet, but no sugar.

So removing all of the sugar from your house does not mean you will never have anything that tastes good again. There are plenty of foods that taste good *and* are good for you. You've just never eaten them before.

So study more about the negative effects of sugar, understand the commitment you are making, gather around others who are making a similar commitment, arm yourself for those tempting times when you are out, and remove all temptations from your own home. Do this, and you will start noticing the difference.

I sincerely hope that this book has proven to be informative and helpful. I hope that your life becomes better because you took to heart what I am saying. I honestly believe that we will have a stronger and happier country if we can get off the sugar addiction and onto living healthier, more prosperous lives.

Chapter 10: The Dare

In this book, I've tried to take the topic of sugar and create a very simple and easy to understand explanation of why you should take *The Dare*. The whole book revolves around this one simple thing . . . take *The Dare*. It is one thing to know something, but it is entirely a different thing to experience it for yourself.

My challenge to each one of you is to take one short month (four weeks to be exact) out of your life to change your diet. This is just twenty-eight days to live a sugar-free lifestyle, that's it! And why did I make it a month and not just a week? Because it takes about twenty-one days to create a new habit. Up until then, the old habits will not be broken and you will only revert back to them. Of course, this will be harder than cutting out cuss words or soap operas because there is the added burden of addiction. This will be more like cutting out smoking. But believe me, it can be done. I know that you can and will do it and I can't wait to see you benefit greatly from it!

**

THE DETAILS—KEEPING IT SIMPLE

Though I can sometimes take something simple and make it complicated, I generally have a unique ability to take things that are complicated and make them nice and simple. I've worked hard at making *The Dare* as simple as possible for everyone so that you can understand why you are doing it as well as what you need to do. I have provided you with a seven-day plan to get you started on your way and to help you kick start the remaining twenty-one days.

Here is a list of what we have provided for you:

Appendix A — I started off by giving you a grocery list for the first seven days. My recommendation would be to just take this book with you and buy what is on the list, even if you don't know what you are going to do with it. Why? Because you will be using them within a week. Don't forget, this will be your food that you eat this week. You are not adding to your grocery bill, this *is* your grocery bill. If you would rather just use the list to help you make your own plan that will work just as well. After all, the main point is to go without refined sugar, not to keep to my specific eating plan.

Appendix B — I have provided for you a daily breakdown of your meals for the first seven days. In this breakdown, I have given you exactly what you should eat for breakfast, lunch, and dinner as well as for snacks in between meals. If you don't like what I've given you to eat, no worries, I've also included a few other meal and snack ideas in Appendix C.

Appendix C — For those of you who would rather have the liberty to make your own meal plan, I've comprised a list of some further options for you. I've broken them down into meal types — breakfast, lunch, dinner, and snacks. If you are like my family, we have breakfast for dinner all the time. It's funny though, we never eat dinner for breakfast. I wonder why. I've also provided some recipes to help you begin to create new favorite recipes.

Appendix D — Allow me to gloat for a minute. I believe that this is a great section. My wife and I have compiled a list of tips that we have learned along our own journey. Some of these I've learned through books, some from other people, and some through trial and error. But read through them. I hope they can help you to feel better and live better and longer.

**

HABITS

Before you go off on your twenty-eight-day journey, I wanted to mention a few things. If I have discovered anything in my life, I have discovered that human beings hate change, me included. Just try changing something from your daily, morning routine. Try putting your left shoe or your left pant leg on first (or vice versa) when you get dressed in the morning. Maybe switch around your schedule. Try eating breakfast before you take a shower, or go to bed one or two hours earlier so you can get up one or two hours earlier. See how much you resist the change. We are all creatures of habit. Change is hard for us because we get comfortable where we are. And the longer we go without changing-up things, the harder it is when things do change, as they always do. A good example is getting married. I've always heard that it is harder to get married when you are older than when you are younger because your lifestyle habits have been solidified. I have seen that first hand in the few people who did get married later in life. They always worked out fine; there was just a longer adjustment period.

But habits can be wonderful things when they are healthy for you. They can also be horrible things when they are not good for you. The habit of regular exercise or positive association is a great habit to have, but the habit of lying or cheating is not. It is interesting to study the most successful people in life. In whatever area that they were successful in, whether it be in family, finances, faith, etc., if you look closely, they had healthy habits in that area. On the flip side, the people who have always struggled have bad habits in the areas they struggled in. Eating refined sugar daily is a habit, and a habit that is unhealthy and needs to be changed. *The Dare* is an attempt to help you make that change before this habit causes damage, which it inevitably is doing and probably doing right now. Don't wait to start. Start as soon as possible. Even if you start and fail, just start again. It is the end result that we are looking for, not a struggle-free attempt. This will take effort, and it will take making and keeping a decision. But now is the time to break the habit. There is a good quote that says, "The chains of habit are too light to be felt until they are too heavy to be broken." How true that is.

**

MONEY

Some of you might say, "I'm on a tight budget right now. I don't have the money!" I can understand what you are saying, and this is a valid concern. I felt the same when I first had to consider changing my diet. However, I have actually found this not to be the case.

Studies show that a large portion of our refined sugar intake comes from our beverages—sodas, sweetened coffees, sports energy drinks, etc. Most people that I talk to who say they don't have enough money are typically drinking some sort of sweet beverage during the day. Do you stop by the local coffee shop regularly? Do you buy sodas, energy drinks, sweet tea, etc.? Living a sugar-free lifestyle is not about adding things to your diet (costing you money) as much as it is taking them away. If you feel that in order to eat sugar-free you will be spending more money than you have, then just try cutting out the sugar beverages for twenty-eight days and drinking water. Not only will you gain the health benefits, but you will also *save* money.

In reality, however, when you balance out the cost of buying foods without sugar and the health benefits, in many cases it will balance out. Aside from the money you will save by cutting out the sugary drinks, if you are suffering from allergies, asthma, or any other chronic illness, how much money are you spending on over-the-counter medication? Have you ever considered this as part of your grocery budget? What about all of those doctor bills because you got the flu because your immune system was lowered by your sweet diet? How much money is spent in your household on pain medication—acetaminophen, ibuprofen, aspirin, etc., from the headaches you've been getting? I don't know everyone's particular situation and whether refined sugar was the cause of it. But more often than not, I would guess that money is being spent on treating illnesses caused by the very habit that is "too expensive" to quit. Think about that. And if this is true for you, it is time to break the chains!

But I'll even go further than this. Even if eating healthy didn't balance out financially with your food and medical bills, what about other areas of your life that are habits that you could cut out? Do you have cable or satellite TV? Do you spend money on concerts or going to sports games? What about eating out; is that a regular occurrence in your household? I'm not saying that these things are not good and that you should never have any fun. What I'm saying is that if you are suffering from a chronic disease that you could possibly eliminate or significantly improve, yet you are choosing not to because you would rather spend your money on entertainment, then I think you should re-examine your priorities. There is nothing worse than losing your health; just ask someone suffering from cancer, osteoporosis, or arthritis. If you are saying that you don't have the money to eat healthy food but are spending your money on other things, you might want to consider add ignoring the truth to your list of unhealthy habits, because you are fooling yourself.

And let me add one more thing about the cost of eating healthy foods, specifically pertaining to cutting out sugar. Even if you decide not to take *The Dare*, you are still going to pay the price . . . at some point. If you don't prioritize your money, time, and efforts on this, you will be giving your money, time, and efforts later when you are going to the doctor, trying to figure out why your joints are aching, why your bones became brittle and broke, why your cholesterol levels are high, why you are so fatigued all the time, why you are having to get pumped full of poisonous chemotherapy "medicines," and why you are being forced to take insulin to regulate your blood sugar. In all reality, the price that you will pay to make this change now by taking *The Dare* is far less than the price you will pay if you do not.

So here is what I want you all to do . . . don't think about taking *The Dare*. Don't wait. Don't debate with yourself. Like the Nike slogan a few years back, *Just Do It!* Go out now, taking your grocery list with you and get what you need. Start *now!*

Appendix A: The Grocery List

This list will supply what you need for the snacks and meals listed in Appendix B. This will get you through the first seven days of your thirty-day sugar-free journey. The recipe quantities are what we would make for our family of six for a meal. Much of what you purchase will last beyond that first week and be used during the rest of the month. In Appendix D "Dietary Tips," there is a list of other foods you may want to stock in your pantry for the month.

Fruits/Vegetables:

- Veggies you like to eat raw (carrots, celery, etc.)
- Dip for veggies (sugar-free)
- Salad-makings (tomatoes, avocado, bell pepper, etc.)
- Spinach for salads
- Apples (tart for a recipe, your favorite for snacking)
- Tomatoes
- Berries
- Celery
- Raisins
- Favorite fruit for snacks
- Grapes
- One red and one yellow bell pepper
- Five medium onions
- Two 6 oz cans tomato paste
- One 28 oz can Cento Italian Style Whole Peeled Tomatoes
- One 16 oz can diced tomatoes
- Two 16 oz cans red kidney beans
- One can beans of choice for nachos (refried or black beans)
- Scallions
- Mushrooms
- Black olives

- Prepackaged fruit with no sugar added (applesauce)
- 1 cup frozen peas
- One carrot
- Fresh ginger

Meat/Cheese/Dairy:

- Two dozen eggs (free range/hormone-free)
- Cheese (for snacks)
- Two bags of pre-shredded cheese
- Parmesan cheese
- Cottage cheese
- Plain, sugar-free yogurt
- Cream cheese
- Chicken Breasts (boneless, skinless)
- Almond Milk
- Deli turkey for sandwiches
- Walnuts or almonds
- Chicken for chicken salad (1-2 large cans or 1-2 skinless breasts)
- 3 lb chicken breasts
- 3 lb of ground meat (chili and nachos — we use turkey)
- Sour cream

Breads/Carbohydrates

- Brown rice
- Sugar-free whole wheat bread (pay attention, most breads that say "whole wheat" are only partially)
- Woven wheat crackers
- Whole wheat tortillas (sugar-free)
- Blue corn chips (for snacks and for nachos for dinner one night)
- Sugar-free cereal (cheerios, granola)
- Plain oatmeal
- Whole wheat English muffins and bagels
- Ezekiel bread (frozen health food section)
- Whole wheat flour
- 6 oz whole wheat spaghetti

- One package whole wheat pasta of your choice
- One to two packages whole wheat tortillas

Others:

- Sugar-free peanut butter
- All fruit
- Hummus
- Whole wheat pita chips
- Salsa/pico de gallo
- Guacamole
- Salt
- Cinnamon
- Yeast
- Nutmeg
- Sugar-free mayo (Duke's yellow label is one of the few that is sugar − free)
- Mustard
- Stevia
- Agave nectar
- Olive oil
- Cumin
- Teriyaki sauce
- Chili powder
- Garlic powder
- Louisiana hot sauce
- Lemon juice
- Lime juice
- Celery seeds
- Minced garlic
- Sweet pickles
- Fresh ground pepper
- Basil
- Rosemary
- Parsley
- Cilantro
- Red pepper

- Seasoned salt
- Taco seasoning mix
- Taco sauce
- Oregano
- Onion powder
- Sesame oil
- Sea salt

Appendix B: The Seven-Day Meal Plan

* When you see an asterisk, you will find a recipe for this in Appendix C.

Day 1/Monday

BREAKFAST:
One to two pieces of cinnamon raisin Ezekiel bread (frozen section of grocery), toasted with butter and a piece of fruit

SNACK 1:
Raw veggies — carrots, celery, peppers, tomatoes, etc., with a sugar-free or no added sugar dip

LUNCH: Spinach salad with chicken (we use grilled chicken from dinner the night before. Marinade recipe included in recipe section). Add veggies of your choice and eat with woven wheat crackers or some whole wheat bread. Add a piece of fruit or handful of nuts.

SNACK 2:
Smiles (a snack our kids love): Put sugar-free peanut butter on one side of an apple slice. Put four to five raisins on the peanut butter on the edge closest to the skin. Put a second slice on top. The skin is the lips and the raisins look like teeth! ☺

DINNER:
Chili* and a piece of whole wheat bread* fresh from your bread maker

NOTES:
_____
_____
_____
_____
_____
_____
_____
_____
_____

Day 2/Tuesday

BREAKFAST:
A sugar-free, whole wheat English muffin with butter, an egg, and a piece of fruit

SNACK 1:
Frogs on a log (great for kids): celery with sugar-free peanut butter spread on it, then add raisins. Substitute almond butter in case of a peanut allergy.

LUNCH:
Chicken salad* sandwich on whole wheat bread, in whole wheat pita pockets, or with woven wheat crackers, with a piece of fruit and some cut up raw veggies

SNACK 2:
Cheese and crackers: For those not cutting out dairy, white cheese (yellow cheese is dyed) with Triscuits. Many whole wheat crackers that are on the market are actually bleached white flour and have added sugar.

DINNER:
Stir fried rice* is a great "one-pot" dinner!

NOTES:
_____
_____
_____
_____
_____
_____
_____
_____
_____

Day 3/Wednesday

BREAKFAST:
Oatmeal (not the pre-packaged, flavored kind as this has a *lot* of sugar). You can flavor it many ways. Our favorite is with cinnamon, butter, raisins, or cut-up apples, and a little Stevia. Another option is sugar-free maple syrup (yummy!). Replace some of the water with almond milk to make it creamier and add some protein.

SNACK 1:
Trail Mix (easy to make yourself, and cheaper, by combining your favorite nuts with sugar-free dried fruit like raisins)

LUNCH:
Egg salad* on whole wheat bread with blue corn chips and a piece of fruit or raw veggies

SNACK 2:
Cottage cheese with some diced fruit

DINNER:
Nachos*

NOTES:

_____
_____
_____
_____
_____
_____
_____
_____
_____

Day 4/Thursday

BREAKFAST:
One cup of plain yogurt (with the lowest sugar content). Don't get pre-flavored because they all add sugar. Add Stevia to taste and fresh, cut up fruit. Greek Yogurt is very high in protein. Add a piece of whole grain, sugar-free toast, lightly buttered.*

SNACK 1:
A piece of fruit—apples, pears, bananas, etc. We love to put sugar-free peanut butter on apple slices for a more filling treat.

LUNCH:
Turkey sandwich with tomato and lettuce on whole wheat bread (see tips about mayo and mustard). Make sure you choose sandwich meat with no sugar or corn syrup. It should have 0 g listed. They frequently use sugar as a preservative in meats. If you can find one with no nitrates that's a bonus! Add fruit or raw veggies.

SNACK 2:
Chips and salsa: Use blue corn chips rather than yellow or white corn. Eat them plain or with some sugar-free guacamole, salsa, or pico de gallo. The salsa will have some sugar grams listed from the tomatoes. Just make sure there is no added sugar on the ingredient list. The deli section of your grocery is the best place to find this.

DINNER:
Spaghetti* with a spinach salad

NOTES:
_____
_____
_____
_____
_____
_____
_____
_____
_____

Day 5/Friday

BREAKFAST:
Homemade cinnamon raisin bread* with an egg and cup of fruit

SNACK 1:
Plain yogurt with added berries and Stevia to taste

LUNCH:
The tried and true peanut butter and jelly sandwich. Of course, neither the peanut butter nor the jelly should have refined sugars. Try "all fruit" types of jelly. Add a piece of fruit, blue corn chips, and raw veggies.

SNACK 2:
A piece of fruit

DINNER:
Chicken and vegetable stir fry* with brown rice

NOTES:
_____
_____
_____
_____
_____
_____
_____
_____
_____
_____

Day 6/Saturday

BREAKFAST:
One to two hormone/antibiotic—free eggs, cooked in your way of choice on the stove (cheese optional depending on if you are cutting out dairy). One to two pieces of whole grain, sugar-free toast, lightly buttered and a piece or cup of your favorite fruit

SNACK 1:
Hard-boiled egg: Sprinkle with salt or other seasoning that you like.

LUNCH:
Wrap: turkey or other meat (no added sugar or preservatives) in a whole wheat tortilla (check sugar content). Add tomato, lettuce, sugar-free salad dressing or mayo. Add a piece of fruit and some blue corn chips or woven wheat crackers.

SNACK 2:
Hummus and whole wheat pita chips

DINNER:
Grilled chicken* with garlic pasta* and a salad

NOTES:
_____
_____
_____
_____
_____
_____
_____
_____
_____

Day 7/Sunday

BREAKFAST:
One to two tablespoons of sugar-free peanut butter or almond butter on sugar-free, whole grain toast with a piece of fruit. If you are used to sugary peanut butter, this takes some getting used to, but is great once you're used to it!

SNACK 1:
A piece of fruit

LUNCH:
Apple-walnut turkey sandwich*. Also, an apple and white cheddar sandwich is good too. Add fruit, raw veggies, or chips.

SNACK 2:
Applesauce, mandarin oranges, or diced fruit with no sugar added. Prepackaged has some preservatives.

DINNER:
Quesdillas*

NOTES:

_____
_____
_____
_____
_____
_____
_____
_____
_____

Congratulations! You have now made it through one-fourth of The Dare! Repeat the meals and snacks from this week or come up with your own for the next three weeks to get to the finish line!

Appendix C: Other Meal and Recipe Options

When you see an asterisk, you will find a recipe for this at the end of this Appendix.

BREAKFAST
Recommend: 1 protein + 1 whole grain + 1 fruit

> One to two cups of almond milk to the sugar-free cereal of your choice with cut up berries or a banana. We typically buy Cheerios because it's difficult to find other cereals without sugar. Sometimes, you can find (or make if you are adventuresome) sugar-free granola at a health food market. You can add a small amount of Stevia if you want it sweetened.

> Hard-boiled egg, sliced and laid on buttered toast

> Hard-boiled egg, sliced. Lay slices on a piece of buttered bread and lay a couple slices of cheese on top. Sprinkle with seasoning of choice. Toast for a couple of minutes.

**

SNACKS
Recommend: one to two snacks between meals, depending on your metabolism and the size of the snack. The healthier the snack the longer it will last you. Mixing proteins with complex carbs is a big key to this!

> Nuts — A handful of almonds, walnuts, etc., often hits the spot for a small snack.

> Raisins or other dried fruit with no sugar added (look carefully to be sure).

> Hummus and whole wheat pita chips.

**

LUNCH

Recommend: one main item that combines protein and whole grains + choose one or two fruit or vegetable choices from the snack list. Avoid adding potato chips or other empty carbohydrates to your meal! If you want something more, add Triscuits or blue corn chips to your lunch.

> ➤ Leftovers! Some people aren't big on leftovers but we love taking something yummy from dinner the night before and reheating it for lunch the next day.

**

DINNER

Recommend: 1 Protein + 1 whole grain/complex carbohydrate + 1 vegetable. Feel free to mix and match to your taste!!

> ➤ Homemade pizza* (any family with kids can't never have enough pizza!)

> ➤ Grill it: Toss a couple burgers on the grill. Add some veggies of your choice*. Don't forget to use whole wheat buns and sugar-free ketchup!

> ➤ Chicken fricassee* with red beans* and rice (Puerto Rican style . . . *yum*!)

> ➤ Chicken divan—casserole night!

DESSERTS

Here are some yummy options to have in place of the normal cookies, ice cream, etc.! These will satisfy your sweet tooth without making you feel guilty!

- Hot chocolate*

- Fruit smoothies*

- Slice of whole wheat bread with honey or agave nectar

- Pumpkin pie* for when you just need to bake! ☺

- Pecan pie* just as good as Grandmother's!

- Apple cider

- Cinnamon applesauce*

Appendix C continued . . . RECIPES

Applesauce, Homemade!

Ingredients:

> ➢ A dozen or more of your favorite apples (we love using Honeycrisp for the sweetness).
> ➢ Water
> ➢ Cinnamon
> ➢ Stevia or agave nectar

Directions:
Peel, core, and chop apples into small pieces. Put apples in crock-pot on low for 8-10 hours or high for 4-5 hours. You can use more or less apples, depending what your crock-pot can hold. Add 1 cup of water to start then check hourly to see if your applesauce needs more liquids. About 1 hour before your applesauce is finished, add ¼ cup cinnamon and sweetener if desired (taste first to see if sweetener is needed — we usually don't add any!). Taste in about 30 minutes to decide if you want more cinnamon or sweetener. *Note:* The sweeter the apples, the sweeter the applesauce! Honeycrisp apples are a good one. Granny Smith apples make a nice tart applesauce.

Apple-Walnut Turkey Sandwiches

Ingredients:

> ➢ ¾ cup sugar-free mayo
> ➢ ¼ cup chopped celery
> ➢ ¼ cup sugar-free, dried fruit (such as raisins)
> ➢ ¼ cup chopped walnuts, toasted (optional)
> ➢ 1 medium tart apple, chopped
> ➢ Deli turkey (sugar-free, preservative-free)
> ➢ Lettuce
> ➢ Whole grain bread

Directions:
Combine all ingredients except lettuce, turkey, and bread. Put turkey on bread and top with mixture, lettuce and second piece of bread. Makes four sandwiches.

Chicken Divan

Ingredients:

- ➤ Two 10 oz packages frozen broccoli spears
- ➤ 1 to 2 pounds of chicken, boneless
- ➤ Two 10 ¾ oz cans condensed cream of chicken soup
- ➤ 1 cup sugar-free mayonnaise
- ➤ 1 ½ tsp lemon juice
- ➤ ¾ tsp curry powder
- ➤ ½ cup sharp cheddar cheese, grated
- ➤ ¾ cup whole wheat bread crumbs

Directions:
Cook broccoli and drain. Cut chicken into bite sized pieces and stir fry. Put broccoli in bottom of baking dish and cover with chicken. Combine soup, mayo, lemon juice, and curry powder in a mixing bowl. Pour over chicken. Top with grated cheese and bread crumbs. Bake at 400 degrees 20-30 minutes. Serve over brown rice. Serves four to six.

Chicken Fricassee

Ingredients:

- ➤ 3 lbs chicken, cut in bite-sized chunks
- ➤ 1 tbsp salt
- ➤ ½ tsp marjoram/oregano
- ➤ 2 cloves, minced garlic
- ➤ ¼ tsp pepper
- ➤ 2 tbsp vinegar
- ➤ ¼ lb chopped ham
- ➤ 3 oz sliced onions

- ➤ 1-2 green bell peppers
- ➤ 1 bay leaf
- ➤ ½ cup olive oil
- ➤ ½ cup tomato sauce
- ➤ 1 lb pared, quartered potatoes
- ➤ ½ cup olives
- ➤ 1 tsp capers

Directions:

Mix salt, marjoram, garlic, pepper, and vinegar in bowl. Rub chicken. If using more than 1 lb of chicken, you may have to make more of the marinade. Allow to marinate in the fridge for 3 hours. Place chicken in large pot with all ingredients *except* potatoes, olives, and capers. Stir and cover, cooking over low heat until chicken is tender. Stir two to three times while cooking. When chicken is tender, add olives, capers, and potatoes. Cook until potatoes are tender. Serve with red beans and rice.

Chicken Salad Colorful

Ingredients:

- ➤ 2 cups cooked chicken breasts, cubed
- ➤ ¼ cup chopped celery
- ➤ ¼ cup golden raisins
- ➤ ¼ cup dried cranberries (no sugar added)
- ➤ ¼ cup sliced almonds
- ➤ ¾ cup sugar-free mayo or sugar-free salad dressing
- ➤ 2 tbsps chopped red onion
- ➤ ¼ teaspoon salt (optional)
- ➤ ¼ teaspoon pepper

Directions:

Combine all ingredients. Put ½ cup into each whole wheat pita pocket.

Chicken Salad Made Easy

Ingredients:

- 1-2 cans chicken, drained, or 1-2 cooked chicken breasts, cubed
- ½ cup or more of chopped grapes or 1 medium tart apple, chopped
- ¼ cup sliced almonds
- Sugar-free mayo to desired consistency
- Cumin to taste

Directions:

Combine all ingredients in a bowl and mix. This is an easy recipe to make in large amounts to have extra! Play with the seasonings and add what you like (like celery salt, a little agave nectar for sweetness, or poppy seeds).

Chicken and Vegetable Stir Fry

Ingredients:

- 1 lb chicken, cubed and marinated in teriyaki sauce
- 1 red bell pepper
- 1 yellow bell pepper
- 1 medium onion

Directions:

Brown chicken in teriyaki sauce. Add bell pepper and onion and cook until onion is translucent. Serve over brown rice. Note: For best results with brown rice, use rice cooker or follow directions on back exactly. It's very easy to make.

Chili

Ingredients:

- 1 lb ground turkey or beef
- 1 medium onion
- 2 tsp salt

- ➢ Two 6 oz cans tomato paste
- ➢ Two 16 oz cans red kidney beans
- ➢ 1 ½ oz chili powder garlic powder to taste
- ➢ Louisiana Hot Sauce to taste
- ➢ Water

Directions:
Brown meat in frying pan. Transfer to large pot. Use small amount of oil from meat to cook onion until clear. Add olive oil if needed. Add onion to pot with all other ingredients. Simmer 2-2 ½ hours. This is an easy recipe to modify to your tastes!

Cinnamon Raisin Bread

Ingredients:

- ➢ 1 cup water
- ➢ ¼ cup olive oil
- ➢ ½ cup agave nectar
- ➢ 2 ½ cups whole wheat flour (if you have a wheat grinder use hard white wheat for your flour)
- ➢ 1 tsp salt
- ➢ 1 tsp cinnamon
- ➢ ½ tsp nutmeg
- ➢ 1 ¾ tsp fast rise or bread maker yeast
- ➢ 1/3 cup raisins

Directions:
Put ingredients in bread-maker pan in order. Choose whole wheat selection and medium-sized loaf. You can double the recipe if you only make the dough in the bread maker. Once the dough is finished, divide in half and form into a loaf shape. Place in two oiled, floured loaf pans. Bake in preheated oven for 30 minutes at 350 degrees. For fun, divide dough in thirds and stretch/roll them into "snakes." Place on oiled cookie sheet and pinch one end of the three "snakes" together. Braid and pinch other end together. Bake 30 minutes at 350 degrees.

Egg Salad

Ingredients:

- 6 eggs, hard boiled and chopped
- Sugar-free mayo to desired consistency
- Yellow, non-spicy mustard, to taste
- Celery seeds, to taste
- 1-2 stalks of celery, chopped *or* 1-2 sweet pickles chopped

Directions:
Combine all ingredients.

Fruit Smoothies

Ingredients:

- ½ ripe avocado (replaces the dairy to give thickness)
- 1 c frozen fruit of choice (peaches or strawberries)
- 1-2 bananas, chopped
- ½ cup apple juice or water
- Dozen or so fresh strawberries or equivalent amount of other berries
- ½ ripe pineapple

Directions:
Combine all ingredients in blender and blend until all chopped up. Makes one blender-full.

Garlic Pasta

Ingredients:

- 6 oz whole wheat spaghetti noodles, cooked
- 3 cloves garlic, minced
- Fresh ground pepper
- 3 tbsp olive oil
- Basil, rosemary, parsley, or other herbs to taste
- Parmesan cheese

Directions:
Slightly stir fry garlic if desired (the more raw it is, the more flavorful). Mix garlic, pepper, olive oil, and herbs with hot spaghetti. Serve topped with parmesan cheese.

Grilled Chicken Marinade

Ingredients:

- ➤ 1 ½ lbs boneless, skinless chicken breasts
- ➤ 1/3 cup olive oil
- ➤ ¼ cup lime or lemon juice
- ➤ 1 tsp garlic powder
- ➤ 1 tsp cilantro
- ➤ ¼ tsp ground cumin
- ➤ ¼ tsp ground red pepper
- ➤ ¼ tsp seasoned salt

Directions:
In medium-sized bowl, mix olive oil with juice and all seasonings. Add chicken. Coat well and refrigerate 30 minutes or more. Grill 10 minutes or until cooked through.

Grilled Vegetables

Directions:
Grilling vegetables is easy, so pick your favorite and enjoy! Here are some tips to help. The general rule is to cut the vegetables into pieces that will cook quickly and evenly. All pieces should be of consistent thickness and no more than about ¾ to 1 inch thick. Cut off ends of vegetables like asparagus, carrots, etc. For each vegetable listed, soak in cold water for about 30 minutes after cutting to keep them from drying out. Pat dry, then brush lightly with olive oil to prevent sticking. *Do not overcook!* For smaller vegetables, you may want to try using a grilling basket to keep them out of the fire.

➢ **Asparagus:** Place on grill, turning every minute. Remove when tips start to turn brown. You can add some extra flavor to asparagus by mixing a little sesame oil in the olive oil before you brush them.

➢ **Bell Peppers:** Cut through the middle of the pepper top to bottom. Remove stems, seeds and whitish ribs. Brush lightly with oil and grill for 2-3 minutes on each side

➢ **Chili Peppers:** Brush with oil. Grill whole on each side, 2-3 minutes. To reduce the heat, cut off the stems and pull out the seeds.

➢ **Corn on the cob:** Gently pull back the husks but don't remove. Remove the silk and cut off the very end. Soak in cold water for about 30 minutes. Dry and brush with butter. Fold the husks back down and tie or twist the ends. Place on grill for about 5-7 minutes. Turn to avoid burning.

➢ **Eggplant:** Cut lengthwise for smaller eggplants or in disks top to bottom for larger eggplants. Grill 2-3 minutes.

➢ **Garlic:** Take whole bulbs and cut off the root end. Brush with olive oil and place cut side down over a hot fire. Grill garlic bulbs for about 10 minutes or until the skin is brown.

➢ **Mushrooms:** Rinse off dirt and pat dry. Brush with oil and grill. 4-5 minutes for small mushrooms, 6-8 minutes for the larger ones. Use a grill basket or topper for small mushrooms if necessary.

➢ **Onions:** Remove skin and cut horizontally about ½ inch thick. Brush with oil and grill 3-4 minutes.

➢ **Potatoes**: There are many ways to grill potatoes. You can do them whole for a baked potato or cut into wedges. For wedges, brush with olive oil, and grill until browned. For a whole potato, wash thoroughly and dry. Rub with oil then cut slit in potato and put butter, a chunk of sliced onion or garlic cloves, and sprinkle oregano or any seasoning you like. Wrap in aluminum foil and grill 35-40 minutes, turning occasionally. Great camping recipe (just toss in fire for 30-45 minutes).

➢ **Tomatoes**: (Yes, I know, technically a fruit) Cut in half, top to bottom. Brush with a light coating of oil and grill cut side down 2-3 minutes.

➢ **Zucchini and Small Squash:** Slice ½ inch thick. Brush with oil and grill 2-3 minutes per side. Small squash can be cut down the middle and grilled in halves.

Hot Chocolate

Ingredients:

- ➤ Almond milk
- ➤ Unsweetened cocoa
- ➤ Stevia

Directions:

Hot chocolate is easy to cook in a pot on the stove or in the crock-pot for large quantities. Mix ¼ cup of cocoa per 4 cups of almond milk. Once it's heated, taste to see if you want to add more cocoa. Sweeten with Stevia to taste. I would start with 1 tbsp per 4 cups almond milk and go from there. If you prepare it in a crock-pot, mix 3 hours ahead and cook on high for approximately 1 hour then turn to low until ready to serve.

Nachos Gonzo Grande

Ingredients:

- ➤ 1 bag of blue corn chips
- ➤ 1 can of refried beans, refried black beans, or plain black beans
- ➤ Shredded cheese
- ➤ 1 lb ground turkey or beef
- ➤ 1 onion
- ➤ Taco seasoning mix
- ➤ Taco sauce or salsa
- ➤ Guacamole
- ➤ Sour cream
- ➤ Any other toppings you like (jalapeños, black olives, etc.)

Directions:

Cook meat over medium heat until cooked through. Add onions and cook until translucent. Add packet of taco seasoning mix and follow directions on the packet. Spread whole bag of nachos on a cookie sheet (can use less — this feeds our family of six). When meat is finished, spread over chips. Add desired amount of beans. Sprinkle with cheese. Add taco sauce or salsa on top. Bake at 375 degrees until cheese is melted. Serve with guacamole and sour cream on the side. This is a family favorite our kids request over and over! Very easy to make!

Pecan Pie

Pie Crust, Homemade

Ingredients:

- ➢ 2 cups flour (if you can used freshly milled flour, it is all the better)
- ➢ 1 tsp salt
- ➢ 2/3 cups plus 2 tbsp butter
- ➢ 7 tbsp cold water

Directions:
Combine the flour and salt in a large bowl. Cut in the butter. Add water and mix. If the dough is too wet, add a little more flour until the right consistency. Divide the dough into half and roll out on a floured surface. Makes 1 double pie crust.

The Pecan Pie Filling

Ingredients:

- ➢ 2 cups liquid sweetener—we use 1 cup agave nectar and 1 cup sugar free maple syrup.
- ➢ 3 large eggs
- ➢ 1/3 cup butter—room temp
- ➢ 1 cup pecans—broken
- ➢ 1 tsp vanilla extract
- ➢ 1 tsp salt
- ➢ 1 uncooked pie crust

Directions:
Preheat the oven to 350 degrees. Roast the pecans in a dry skillet over medium heat for 5 minutes then set aside. Gently boil the liquid sweetener in a pan for 10 minutes then remove from heat. Lightly beat the eggs, then gradually pour

into the heated liquid sweetener. Be careful to continue mixing to keep the eggs from scrambling. Cut the butter into little chunks and add to the mixture while continuing to beat the egg and sweetener mixture. Stir in the vanilla extract. Lay roasted pecans on uncooked pie crust and pour the mixture over the pecans. Put the pie on a cookie sheet and place in the oven, being careful not to spill. Bake for about 30 minutes, then add a pie crust shield and bake for another 30 minutes. The total cook time is around one hour. You can test the pie by putting a knife into the center of the pie. If the filling sticks to the knife, put it back in for another few minutes. If the knife comes out clean, it is done. Cool pie on a wire rack before eating.

Pizza Crust (1 medium pizza):

Ingredients:

- 5/8 cup hot water
- ¼ cup milk
- 1 tbsp olive oil
- ½ tbsp agave nectar or honey
- 1 tbsp instant yeast
- 2-2 ½ cups hard white wheat freshly milled or whole wheat flour
- 1 tsp salt
- ½ tsp gluten (optional)

Directions:
You have several options for making the dough.

- *By hand*: If you choose to make the dough by hand, you can easily double the recipe to make two pizzas. Stir ingredients together. Kneed just slightly, about 5 minutes, to make a smooth ball. Let rise until double. Turn onto floured surface and divide in half. Roll onto greased pizza pans. Cover with tomato sauce. Sprinkle with oregano. Add desired toppings. Bake at 400 degrees 20-25 minutes.
- *Bread maker*: Put ingredients in your bread maker, liquids first and yeast last. Put on the dough setting. Start with 2 cups of flour, then check every so often as it mixes and add more if the dough seems to be sticky. The bread machine will let you know when the dough is ready.

> *Food processor or mixer with dough attachment*: If you use either of these, put all ingredients together and let mix until it makes a smooth ball. Put in oiled bowl and let rise until double. Continue as above.
> *Freezing for later*: Roll out the finished dough on pizza pans. Let sit for 10-15 minutes. Bake at 400 degrees for 10-12 minutes. Cool and wrap in plastic wrap. Freeze until ready to use. When ready to eat, add toppings and bake about 15 minutes.

Pumpkin Pie (no gluten, dairy, sugar)

Ingredients:

> 3 eggs
> ¼ cup water
> 1 can pumpkin puree
> ¾ cup coconut milk, lite (almond milk?)
> 15 drops stevia liquid
> 1/6 cup honey or agave nectar
> ¼ tsp sea salt
> ½ tsp nutmeg
> ¼ tsp allspice
> ¼ tsp ginger root
> 1/8 tsp cloves
> Unbaked pie shell (see "pie crust, homemade" on previous page)

Directions:
Mix all wet ingredients in mixing bowl. Add dry ingredients and stir with whisk until well mixed. Pour mixture into unbaked pie shell. Pie crust recipe on previous page. Bake at 425 degrees for 15 minutes. Lower temperature to 350 degrees and bake for 35-40 more minutes.

Quesadillas

Ingredients:

> One or two packages whole wheat tortillas (depends on how many you want to make) butter shredded cheese (we buy the "Mexican

Mix" pre-shredded) scallions or a small onion, chopped and lightly sautéed mushrooms, sliced and lightly sautéed black olives, chopped salsa taco sauce sour cream
- Any other toppings you like (chicken, grilled veggies, black beans)

Directions:
Melt butter to grease large skillet. Turn heat to medium. Lay a tortilla in skillet until heated on one side and barely crispy. Set aside and cook another tortilla the same. Flip second tortilla over (add more butter as needed). Sprinkle with a layer of cheese and add desired toppings (scallions/onions, mushrooms, black olives, chicken, etc.). Sprinkle another layer of cheese and cover with first tortilla, cooked side down. Let cook until cheese is mostly melted. Flip over to cook other side (the more toppings you put in, the harder to flip!). Once all cheese is melted and tortilla is cooked to desired crispiness, put quesadilla on a plate and let cool a moment. Cut into eight pieces with a pizza cutter. Serve with sour cream and salsa. Repeat as many times as your family will eat! Our family of six usually polishes off four to six of them for dinner.

Red Beans and Rice

Ingredients:

- Two cans of red kidney beans
- 1 can full of water
- 1 green bell pepper
- 2 capfuls of vinegar
- 1 tbsp olive oil
- One 15 oz can tomato sauce
- 2 tsp paprika

Directions:
Mix all ingredients in a large pot. Bring to a boil, lower heat, and cook for 1 hour. Serve over brown rice.

Spaghetti

Ingredients:

- ➢ One package of your favorite shape whole wheat pasta, cooked
- ➢ One 28 oz can Cento Italian style whole peeled tomatoes
- ➢ One 16 oz can diced tomatoes
- ➢ One 16 oz can water
- ➢ 1 tbsp oregano
- ➢ 1 tbsp garlic powder
- ➢ 1 tbsp onion powder
- ➢ 1 medium onion
- ➢ 1 cup parmesan cheese, shredded
- ➢ 2 tsp basil
- ➢ 1 tsp minced garlic
- ➢ 1 lb ground turkey or beef

Directions:

Brown meat and put in large sauce pot. Sauté onion in oil from the meat until translucent. Add minced garlic. Gently brown. Add to large sauce pot. Add tomatoes and all other ingredients, including parmesan cheese, to pot. Bring to a boil. Reduce heat and simmer 20-30 minutes.

Stir fried rice

Ingredients:

- ➢ 4 cups cooked brown rice
- ➢ ¼-½ lb chicken breasts, cubed and stir fried *or* smoked sausage
- ➢ 2 eggs, scrambled and chopped (optional)
- ➢ Sesame oil dash sea salt
- ➢ 1 cup frozen green peas, thawed (optional)
- ➢ 1 carrot, chopped in small cubes
- ➢ ½ onion, chopped *or* 4 scallions, chopped
- ➢ 1 cup chopped mushrooms
- ➢ Fresh ginger to taste

Directions:
Stir fry the meat in small sauté pan until done. Set aside. Heat sesame oil over medium heat in wok or large sauté pan. Add onions, mushrooms, carrots, peas, and dash of salt. Sauté approximately 5 minutes (carrots should still be slightly crunchy). Lower heat and add ginger. Sauté 1-2 more minutes. Add cooked rice, scrambled egg, and meat. Mix well. This recipe can be easily tailored to your tastes! It can also be simplified.

o   Simplified variation: Heat sesame oil in large stir fry pan. Add ½ bag of mixed, frozen peas and chopped carrots. When heated through, add rice, meat, and egg, if desired. Season with salt, pepper, and/or soy sauce.

Whole Wheat Bread

Ingredients:

➤   1 cup water
➤   ¼ cup olive oil
➤   ¼ cup agave nectar or honey
➤   2 ½ cups whole wheat flour (if you have a wheat grinder use hard white wheat for your flour)
➤   1 tsp salt
➤   1 ¾ tsp fast rise or bread maker yeast

Directions:
Put ingredients in bread-maker pan in order. Choose whole wheat selection and medium sized loaf. It will be ready in about 3 ½ hours in bread maker.

o   Note: This bread is even better if you double the recipe and set your bread maker on "dough" setting. When finished, turn out dough on floured surface and divide in half. If it's a bit sticky, just add more flour and knead for a few seconds. Form each half into a loaf shape and place in two oiled, floured loaf pans. Bake at 350 degrees for 30 minutes.

Appendix D: General Dietary Tips

➤ We have listed some ideas for each meal and snack in Appendix E, but they are by no means the only things you can eat. Use these tips to get you started in coming up with healthy foods that you like. You'll be surprised what you can come up with if you try. Also, while it is more expensive to eat healthier, you will find that you actually consume less food because your body is getting the nutrients that it needs.

CHILDREN AND SUGAR:

➤ If you have children and you plan to do *The Dare* as a family, you're doing a great thing for them! You will need to be prepared for some resistance (our kids really push back at times, and at others it's no big deal). Here are a few things you can do to help.

➤ Discuss and explain what you are doing no matter how young they are. Let them know what the plan and expectations are in the beginning.

➤ Whenever you go out to eat, even if it's to someone's house, decide ahead of time if you will partake in dessert/sweets, if you'll take your own sugar-free dessert, or if you just say no. Then prepare the kids (and yourself) to resist temptation! We have gone to many birthday parties and just politely said "no thanks" to cake. We try to get our kids to focus on the reason for the occasion rather than the treats.

➤ It's OK to stay home! If your kids are really struggling with the no sugar thing, it's OK not to go to the birthday party or to leave the room during the cake! It's hard to break that addiction, so be understanding while not giving into to the desire.

➤ Prepare the grandparents and others you see frequently and ask them not to offer your kids sweets. It makes it much easier if they know ahead of time. At family events, we always bring something for our family to eat, like a sugar-free apple pie. Beware that your kids aren't the only ones who will resist what you are doing . . . family or friends may not understand what you are doing as well!

➢ Chat with your child's teacher, Sunday school teacher, etc. This has always been a challenge for us. Teachers love to give treats to kids. We began supplying sugar-free treats and small toys for them to give our kids.

➢ Be prepared for surprises. I'm always caught off guard by the waitress who sets mints on the table in front of my kids. The teller who offers a lollipop without asking first. Practice with your kids telling that person "no, thank you." Otherwise, they'll look at you like, "hey, can I eat this?" and you may have to do battle in public!

➢ The bottom line: With kids, it all comes down to how serious you are about cutting out sugar and sticking to whatever guidelines you set up. At one time, our guidelines were that we had a small bit of our candy on Halloween; we could eat one thing at birthdays and Christmas parties, etc. Basically, we were limiting our sugar intake to special occasions. What we noticed was that those occasions were becoming very frequent. So we had a parental powwow and let the kids know we were updating the guidelines. Birthday parties were no longer treat occasions, nor were boy and girl scout celebrations, reading parties at school, etc. Now we have sugary treats on very rare occasions and then in limited amounts. But the guidelines you set up have to fit your family!

GENERAL:

➢ Become a label reader! "Sugar" is not the only ingredient to watch out for: cane juice, molasses, honey, sugar, agave nectar, and corn syrup also. While agave nectar and honey are healthier versions of sugar, they should be used sparingly, especially for those with diabetes or hypoglycemia. I noticed that after putting agave nectar in a cup of tea that I had the same "funny" feeling I get when I've had sugar or honey due to my hypoglycemia.

➢ You should start noticing that most foods have sugar in them, used mostly as a preservative.

➢ Pay attention to your cravings. Your moods can tell you what your body needs. If you are craving sugar, it could mean that your body wants protein. Ever notice that sometimes, a salad just sounds good? Or how about that orange on those summer days? Your body will tell you what it needs.

➢ Eat balanced meals. An "all carbs" diet will lead you down a path of ill health pretty quickly. Make sure you are including a protein, fiber, and essential oils (omega 3), along with your whole grains.

➢ "Daniel Fast" diet plans are a great source of recipes and meal ideas. Some websites to check out are:
  o http://www.jentezenfranklin.org/fasting/danielfast.php
  o http://danielfast.elevationchurch.org/

➢ Avoid micro-waving food. It destroys the nutrients.

SWEETENERS, BEVERAGES, AND CAFFEINE:

➢ Stevia is an herb that can be used as a natural, non-chemical. There are many brands on the market and can come in liquid or powder form. The amount used is very tiny compared to the amount needed for granulated sugar or a sugar substitute. It also should not affect your blood sugar. A great resource is www.cookingwithstevia.com. They have lots of info about the herb as well as recipes!

➢ While we all like variety, our body needs water; it is just a fact. Your body's makeup is 70% water. It is important to drink plenty of it. Many people complain that they don't like to drink water. That's like saying breathing irritates you! Add some juice from a citrus fruit to it and drink it anyway (and no, tea does not count as water!).

➢ Unfortunately, in today's world just drinking out of the tap is not healthy. There are so many chemicals and wastes in our water that we would recommend a good filter for your faucet. It's much more cost effective in the long run than always buying bottled water.

➢ If you can handle cutting out caffeinated beverages during this week, do it! You'll notice even more drastic results. The combination of sugar and caffeine are powerful. Caffeine is a "vasodilator," which means that it makes your veins expand so more blood can move through your system. Unfortunately, when you combine that with sugar, you make an even faster way for the sugar to get in the bloodstream.

➢ Side note: If you are cutting out sugar, please don't replace your soda with diet soda! There are so many negative effects from the ingredients in soda, one major one being women getting osteoporosis in their twenties! Another is symptoms that mimic multiple sclerosis. Just say *no!*

➢ While you're doing this challenge, try to avoid artificial sweeteners as much as you can as well. Some sweeteners actually cause your cells to retain water, others can cause stomach upset. None of them are good for you.

VITAMINS:

➢ If you don't currently take vitamins, please consider supplementing with vitamins. Our food is depleted of many of its nutrients due to processing or being picked before it is ripe. Fruits and vegetables are radiated to keep them from aging too quickly (apples can spend as much as a year in cold storage according to one of our horticulturist friends!). This destroys their nutrients.

➢ Don't just grab some handy brand of vitamins off the store shelf because it is cheap. Research vitamin companies. Look for companies that own their own farms, use natural pesticides rather than chemicals, and make their products from organically grown plants.

➢ If you take nothing else vitamin-wise, consider researching and finding a really good multivitamin, probiotics (what's in yogurt is *not* adequate!), and digestive enzymes.

➢ If you don't consume fish a couple times a week, you'll also want to consider omega 3's or fish oil as well. This is a great supplement to give your kids especially! Helps with brain development and focus.

SPECIFIC FOODS:

> Almond milk is a great substitute for milk. Our kids drink it like it's milk (be sure to get unsweetened), and we put it in cereal. Soy milk has been linked to some possible negative side effects and rice milk has a high natural sugar content.

> Almonds: These are the best nut for you to eat. They are the only nut that is alkaline rather than acidic. Diseases live in acidic environments, and we eat a large amount of acidic foods in our society (salt and sodas!). They also neutralize strong flavors in your mouth; so they're great for your breath after a cup of coffee or garlic! Get them raw and unseasoned.

> Avocado is a great substitute for dairy in recipes like smoothies and puddings. You can't taste it at all, and it helps them be creamy and thick!

> Butter: Use regular butter in cooking. It is all-natural and tastes better than the fake stuff. Not to mention, the fake stuff is worse for you than the "real" stuff with all its chemicals.

> Condiments: The only sugar-free mayo that we have found is "Dukes" brand. Most mustards don't have sugar in their ingredients. Ketchup will have to go as they all have added sugar!

> Dairy breaks down into lactose (a sugar) in your body, so try to limit your dairy. When you look at grams of sugar on a food label, you'll see some sugar listed on dairy items (milk, cheese, etc.), even if there is no sugar added.

> Fish: Fish is a great, healthy option for dinner. We don't eat a lot of fish at our house due to picky palates, and since many people don't eat it, we didn't include it in our meal plan. It's a great source of omega 3s, the healthy fatty acid!

> Fruit: Whole fruit is digested differently because it was designed to have the combination of the fiber and sugar. When you remove the fiber (i.e. juice), you are getting pure sugar. So stay away from juice.

Also avoid canned fruit/applesauce, unless they are free from added preservatives or sugar.

➢ Pasta and rice: Most meals could be made healthier simply by changing to whole wheat pasta and brown rice.

➢ Salads: We always use spinach in our salads and romaine on sandwiches. The darker the leaf, the more nutrients, especially vitamin C. Iceberg lettuce is just plain fiber, no nutrients.

➢ Salad Dressings: You will need to make your own vinaigrette dressing for your salads or hunt for a sugar-free dressing. "Walden Farms" is a brand that makes sugar-free, preservative-free salad dressings.

➢ Snacks: We are big believers in small, healthy snacks between meals. This helps your will power immensely if you are dieting or trying a new diet plan for the first time!

DESSERTS:

➢ During this month, you are working to change some eating habits, not going on a diet. One habit many of us in the States have is that dessert is a necessary part of each meal. We all love something sweet, but for the first week, avoid having "dessert." After that first week, try one of the fruit smoothies for a sweet reward for one week of healthy eating!

BREAD

➢ It is very hard to find bread with no sugar in it. Nature's Valley makes a sugar-free, whole wheat bread. Look for whole wheat breads, not bleached or anything else.

➢ Ezekiel bread, found in the freezer section, also does not have sugar in it, as well as being gluten-free. It is great for toast and they make several different kinds.

➢ Honestly, the best way to go is to make your own bread. Make a sugar-free, whole wheat bread. We use a bread maker so it takes very little time and effort to make our bread.

➢ We invested in a wheat grinder. It cost about the same as a really good bread maker. We buy wheat and other grains in bulk (it keeps forever), and it takes about thirty seconds to grind a few cups of flour. This way we are getting the complete nutrients. You can actually buy "white" wheat and make "white bread" that is healthy this way. Check out www.breadbeckers.com for more info on this.

➢ Stay away from store-bought white bread completely. It has no nutritional value *at all* and, as a simple carbohydrate, turns into sugar during digestion.

Other foods you may want to stock during *The Dare*:

—Sugar-free spaghetti sauce
—Sausage (hard to find without sugar as a preservative)
—Dried beans—which you use in any dish.
—Broccoli
—Avocado (healthy fats)
—Frozen vegetables (broccoli, lima beans, peas, etc.)
—Any other fresh fruits and vegetables that you like to eat.
—Curry
—Dill
—Rosemary
—Splenda (though it is a chemical as well and should be used sparingly)
—Butter
—Cottage cheese

Appendix E: Something More Important

All names used in the following stories have been changed to protect the privacy of those mentioned. However, the stories are true to the best of my knowledge and memory.

Knock, knock, knock . . . I heard the light tapping on the back screen door but paid little attention to it. I was busy watching my favorite cartoon, Scooby Doo. I was around eight or nine and loved my TV time. And though I didn't much pay much attention to time, I did pay attention to when it was four o'clock, because that was when Scooby came on!

And this day was no different. I had jumped off the school bus an hour or so earlier and started the walk toward home with my best friend, Ray. We chatted cheerily. When we got closer to our homes, we agreed that Ray was going to stop by his house to check in with Mom and then come over to my house to watch Scooby Doo. We split up and went our separate ways.

After hearing the knock on the door, I heard the old spring on our back screen door creak and my mom say cheerfully, "Oh hey, Ray!" A moment of silence followed and then I heard my mother say in a much more subdued tone, "Tony, could you come here, please." I thought it was a bit strange that she didn't just let him in; Ray was like another son to my parents, and that is what they normally did.

I got up and walked to the backdoor. Standing outside of the door was my friend, pale faced and slump-shouldered. He was standing in the door jam, holding the screen door open as if hesitant to enter. My mother said somberly, "Ray has something he needs to tell you." I look to my friend as the tears began to well up in his eyes. He said, "He's dead."

"Oh" I said and just stood there with an uncomfortable silence between us all. I finally broke the silence saying "Do you want to come in and watch TV?" He said, "OK." So we went into the living room, sat side by side on the couch, and watched Scooby Doo, though neither of us were in the mood, because Ray's little brother had just died.

***

I've focused this entire book on one subject, sugar, and I believe wholeheartedly in everything I've written thus far. However, I also believe that there is something even more important than your physical health and that something is your spiritual health.

I think this is more important, because though your physical health can give you a good life right now, your spiritual health can provide you an eternal life. And after all, which one lasts longer? There have been billions of people who have lived on this earth, all who are now gone. Some lived to a ripe old age, and some didn't even make it to puberty. But if there is one thing is undeniable, it is that everyone dies. That we know this for sure.

There are many things that are uncertain in our lives; we don't know whether it is going to rain tomorrow, we don't know whether or not we'll keep our jobs or lose our business, we don't know if we are going to get in a car accident or not, and we don't know if we are going to have a heart attack or not. But there is one thing that is totally and absolutely certain which no sane person can deny, that one day our hearts will stop beating, our bodies will turn cold, and we will die. It is understandably something that most people hate to think about, but nobody can deny that it is the truth—we all will one day perish from this earth and be no more.

***

Driving Without a Map

So why am I telling you this? Let me tell you a story to illustrate . . .

I have been driving for just over twenty years now. In that time, I've driven cars, haul trucks, boom trucks, vans, backhoes . . . you name it. I think my favorite was the haul truck. Those are the big ones that you find in rock quarries, with the tires that are taller than your average man. I drove one during my college days. But whether I was in the large haul truck, the U-Haul trailer, or just my beat up old Honda, rarely did I ever get into the vehicle where I didn't already know where I was going. When I was in the haul truck, I knew where I had to go to pick up rock and where to go to drop it off. When I get in the car today, I already know what I'm doing and where I'm going. If I didn't, I wouldn't know how to figure out which way to go. Here's the interesting part: we do this while we are driving, so why don't we do the same thing when it comes to living (or driving) our lives. Wouldn't it make sense to think about where we are going or what's going to happen? It is inevitable after all.

Most people I know these days look at me like I'm crazy and morbid to even be thinking about this stuff. They act as if I'm "raining on their parade." "There's plenty of time to think about that junk!" they say. But if I got in the car with them and asked them where we were going, they wouldn't say, "Why worry about that now. I don't like to think about that." No, they would tell me where they were going and how they are going to get there. Or at least they would take the time to look at a map to figure it out. Shouldn't we be doing the same? Shouldn't we be trying to figure out what happens to us after we die? It seems to me that it is the most critical part in figuring out how to live the life we have now!

Think of all the people who have at some point been in your life but who no longer exist on this earth. Death certainly rained on their parade. I would guess that many of them did not plan to die when they did. That is why they should serve as good examples of why we should be thinking about this topic now. In terms of the people in my own life, outside of Ray's brother, I can quickly think of a handful of people whose parade was got wet:

> I had an aunt who I really loved. We were very much alike, so we had a sort of bond between us. When I was about twelve and she was thirty, she began having pains in her abdomen. She went to the doctor and discovered that she had ovarian cancer. At the time, she was recently married; she and her husband were both lawyers with brilliant prospects. They were excited about their future and getting ready to expand their family with kids, only for those dreams to be smashed to pieces with one visit to the doctor. I remember when her doctors told her that she'd never have kids. She was crying, but gave my brother and I big hugs, saying that we were her kids now. She only lived a few months after that.

> I remember my high school class valedictorian, Maya. She was a very intelligent and active person. I knew both Maya and her sister Elizabeth. Maya was in my home room and

her sister, a few years younger, played drums with me in the marching band. I'm sure Maya had lots of plans for the future—husband, kids, etc. But within a year from graduating high school, Maya developed a brain tumor and died. Elizabeth was without a sister.

When I was in college, I played on the drum line. I had a good friend, Charles, who played the quads—that is four drums carried by one person. He loved to play the drums and was naturally very good. But Charles was also good at football and had dreams of being a walk-on on the football team. At the beginning of my sophomore year and Charles's junior year, Charles did not stay with band but instead participated in the walk-on tryouts held around the same time as band camp. Apparently, he was doing pretty well because we were getting word while at camp about his great chances of getting on the team. I was pretty excited about knowing someone on the football team. One morning, however, as the heat of the day was just beginning to lay an oppressive blanket over the practice fields, the team took a break from running drills to cool off and get some water. As they were getting back up and heading onto the field, Charles fell flat on his face and died within minutes. You see, Charles had a hole in his heart that he didn't even know was there. There was something about the exertion on the field that made his heart stop, killing him that day. He was barely twenty. I still remember going to the funeral. I got there late as I couldn't find the place. But as I arrived, I remember hearing his mother's cries of pain and sorrow from the parking lot. She was literally wailing. See, Charles was the son everybody loved. He was so full of life. He just had that sparkle in his eyes.

I could go on and on with stories from my own experiences about the death of people in my own life. But what about the one's in yours? If anything, these stories should point to the fact that you never know when your time will be up here on earth. We make plans for our futures, but in reality we don't even know if we'll have tomorrow. The book of James says:

"Now listen, you who say, 'Today or tomorrow we will go
to this or that city, spend a year there, carry on business and
make money.' Why, you do not even know what will happen
tomorrow. What is your life? You are a mist that appears for a
little while and then vanishes. Instead, you ought to say, 'If it
is the Lord's will, we will live and do this or that.'"

James was not saying don't make plans, and he definitely was not saying
don't do anything at all. He was just saying trust in God and to live life always
keeping in mind that it will all end one day and that day might be today. He
was saying know where you are going before you get in the car.

This is so important and will affect every decision in your life. It will play a
part in whether you take that new job offer. Though the job will make more
money, you might find that it takes too much time away from family, which
in light of death might seem more important. It will play a part in whether or
not you go out to the bar with your co-workers from the office instead of going
home to your spouse. It will help you decide whether to live a life seeking
money and fame or to seek a life of significance. This doesn't necessarily mean
that you shouldn't have money and fame; only that they are not the most
important focuses in life.

In reality, thinking about your imminent death will affect every aspect of the
life you live. So why would we not think about what will happen to us? It
makes total sense that we do, not to be morbid but to be realistic, even curious.
We should all be seeking this knowledge so we can direct our lives to the end
we want. Stephen Covey, author of *The Seven Habits of Highly Successful People*
put it this way . . ." begin with the end in mind."

***

A sickness

I am very passionate about health. I love being healthy, and more
importantly, I love feeling healthy. But when I look at most people, all I see
is sickness—spiritual sickness. I hear all the talk about the great parties, the
wild events, the unconfined experiences where people are just living up life.
I've been to many of those "wild" parties, especially when I was younger. But
when I look closely at that person talking, I never really see this life they are

"living up." I see moments of fun, craziness, and unbridled pleasure. But in their regular life, in the in-between moments (which is most of the time), I see spiritual sickness.

Do you know what spiritual sickness is? It is a cancer of the soul, an illness of the heart. I'm not talking about the physical pump that beats inside of us. I'm talking about the *spiritual* heart, the heart that rages when we are mad and that aches when we are sad. And just like a physical illness, where the body hurts, a spiritual sickness is where the soul of a person is hurting. Fear, doubt, a weak self-image, depression, anger, hatred, jealousy, immaturity, detachment—these are just a few of the symptoms of a spiritually sick person. Haven't you ever felt that there was something wrong with your life? Has it ever felt shallow to you? Has it felt unstable and unsafe, or worse, unimportant and unsatisfying? That is spiritual sickness and sometimes spiritual death. What we need is spiritual life!

***

The Source of Life

Have you ever looked at an aerial photograph of Egypt? It is quite interesting. For the most part, it is very dry and dusty. But if you take a closer look at the photo, you will see one line of green that almost splits the country in half. Do you know what that line of green is? It is the Nile River; I believe the only river in the world that runs from south to north. And why is it so green? Because of the vegetation that grows and thrives from the Nile's water and nutrients.

So what does the Nile have to do with spiritual sickness? Listen to what the author of this very old Hebrew poem said a long time ago . . . *paraphrased*

> "Good things come to the person who does not walk alongside angry and hurtful people or stand in the way of wrong-doers or associate with people who mock others. This person delights in learning all about God and how and why He created this world and meditates on this knowledge day and night. A person who does this is like a tree planted by a stream of water, which bears its fruit in season and whose leaf does not wither. Whatever this person does prospers.

Not so with the angry and hurtful people! They are like chaff (the inedible part of the wheat plant) that the wind blows away. Therefore, the angry and hurtful people will not do well on Judgment Day, and the wrong-doers will not end up in the same place as the people who strive to do good in life. For God watches over and protects the right-doers, but the wrong-doers will perish."

Psalm 1

I think the message is pretty clear — human beings are like plants that wither and die the farther away they are from their source of life just like the trees and plants that live around the Nile River die the farther they are from water. A spiritually sick person is a person who is far from their source, likely to invite illness, to wither, and eventually to die. The person is not suffering because they are in the harsh environment like the desert; they are suffering because they are far from their source. And what does being far from your source look like? It would be someone who only rarely thinks about who they are and why they were created. It could be someone who rejects altogether the notion that there is a God. It would be someone who can't admit that they don't have total control over their future and who never taps into the reservoir of knowledge of how to live a blessed life on this earth and into eternity by reading the ancient scriptures. I know this concept of a source and needing to be connected to your source must seem foolish to some of you. But just think about it for a moment. Doesn't all of life come from a source and point to a source? Maybe the reason it seems strange is because it has been so long since you've ever thought about it. Sick people often times don't even know that they are sick until it is too late!

***

Brains, Brains!

I absolutely detest horror movies, I always have. When I was in high school, I was pressured into watching the classic horror flick *Night of the Living Dead*. I don't remember much about the plot of the movie if it even had one. But I do have vivid memories of these beings walking around the cemetery, neither dead nor alive. They were zombies, and they would walk around murmuring creepily, "brains, brains, brains" because that's what they wanted to eat (though they were supposed to be dead — go figure).

I mention this because many of us are walking around like zombies and don't even know it. Over time, the hurts and the fears that we have encountered throughout our lives have made us retreat into inner shells, separating us from our source, separating us from others, and even separating ourselves from our own feelings. We feel hollow inside and isolated. On top of that, we try to fill the void in our lives with meaningless pleasures. We become that dead zombie walking around lustfully trying to consume something that won't bring us back to life. Only, instead of saying "brains, brains, brains," we're saying "fun, fun, fun" or "alcohol, alcohol, alcohol," or "sex, sex, sex" . . . you get the idea. These things in themselves are not bad. However, a dependency on them to stay "happy" will never work. It's not brains the zombies need, it is *life*! And it is not these pleasures or diversions that we need; it is our source . . . *life*!

I remember being with my grandfather when he was dying. He had been suffering from the effects of diabetes for a while and eventually died from an infection that started in his lower legs due to the poor circulation common in diabetics. This was about eleven years ago, and I was in my late twenties. I remember getting a chance to say goodbye to him before he slipped into unconsciousness. It all happened pretty quickly at the end. His breathing became shorter and shorter and more strained until finally he took his last breath in, and let it all out in a sort of drawn-out sigh. In that moment, his eyes popped open, and his head fell to the side. He was gone.

We all sat there for what seemed like an eternity, just taking in the fact that he was no longer alive. Then, one by one, the family began getting up, kissing his cheek, and saying goodbye. When I felt it was my turn, I stood up, leaned over my grandfather, and kissed his cheek. As I did this, I was shocked to notice how lifeless his cheek felt. Only a minute ago, I was touching my grandfather's hand, and there was life in it. But now, only minutes later, he didn't feel like a human being, he felt like a dummy. Actually, to be a little more graphic, it felt like the Thanksgiving turkey I get from the store that has thawed out — just a big hunk of meat and bones with skin. It was cold and lifeless. The life was totally gone.

When you see a physically dead person, it is obvious that there is no life in them. It is plain to see. But let me ask you this, have you ever seen a spiritually dead person? I bet you have. They are easy to spot. All you have to do is to just open your eyes. They are everywhere. Oh, it might be difficult to spot them at the football game, or at the party, or anywhere else where their attentions are diverted and they are having fun. But watch how they are in the down times, if they ever allow themselves to have down time. Or watch them in a crisis. You'll see their true selves come out—the fears, the doubts, the anger. It's there. We just live in a society that is good at covering up.

***

We Are All Relational

Did you know that there are orphanages in some countries where there are so many children the workers don't have enough time to hold and nurture the children? It is well known that if you give everything a baby needs—food, water, diaper changes, etc.—but you deny that baby the physical caressing and nurturing that a mother and father provide, that baby will develop at a much slower rate. In many cases, when there is no physical contact outside of the basic needs, the child will become ill or, worse, they lose their will to live, stop eating or drinking, and die. Why does this happen? Because human beings are relational beings.

I believe that most people today are spiritually dead not only because they are distant from their source (their creator) but also because they don't feel important or loved. There is a hole inside, a cancer that is making them spiritually sick and this hole is their lack of relationship with the God in heaven who made them on purpose and who loves them.

Now understand this, I'm not talking about religion. Religion is a man-made structure comprised of people who are all sinners, all hypocrites, all selfish and untrustworthy. There is a definite place for church and a church structure, but I'm talking about religion overall. When it comes to Christianity, most of the worst examples of Christians are Christians themselves. Did you know that going to church will not fill up that hole inside of you; though going to church is a great thing? Did you know that working at a church or even becoming a pastor won't fill it up either, though these are also great things? Not even serving others who have less than you at a soup kitchen or building homes for the poor will fill up this hole inside, though if you are doing these things, keep it up! But why won't they fill up the hole? Because your relationship with your creator is not about what you do. He made you to be his blessed child whom He loves. He made you to be in a *relationship* with Him where you feel so safe, so protected, so loved that you just emanate joy and peace, like the beloved son who lives carefree knowing his father is there to protect and love him.

But most of us don't have a relationship with God. Many of us don't even talk to Him. We feel like God is as close to us as the stars are to the Earth. And that is why we are spiritually sick zombies. I know what it feels like to be spiritually sick. I remember how lost and scared I felt only a few short years ago when I couldn't seem to find a job and money was always short. I remember how I felt when my wife and I saw the child that we wanted to adopt go home to a life of neglect and eventually incurred brain damage due to this neglect. I remember how I felt when my wife so badly wanted to have a child but only had miscarriages. I remember when it felt like the weight of the world was on my shoulders, how I felt that I was just another pawn in the rough game of life, in danger of being cut down by a more powerful bishop or rook at any moment. I felt that I was losing control and that everything was being pulled out of my hands. I was afraid my fears would come true—that maybe I really am a nobody, maybe I don't matter, and maybe I don't have what it takes to make it in this life. I really felt like I was in that desert, far from the waters of the Nile, all alone with no one who even cared. I wanted so badly to discover a different truth, one where I wasn't just a nobody, one where I actually mattered and where I could have hope. But mostly, I just remember wanting to stop being afraid.

If you have picked up this book, you might be feeling that longing in your spirit for something more, something meaningful. I know you were not expecting to pick up a book about health and be hearing all this spiritual stuff. I know that many of you are just waiting for the punch line delivered by some religious fanatical doctrine. The truth is, there is no punch line. There is a sincere desire to help those who are struggling. I want people to first see their sickness and then for them to know the peace that comes through a true faith, despite their current problems in life.

But what about you? Maybe you are in an unhappy marriage where it started off good and life was fun and exciting. But now life hasn't turned out the way you imagined. Now you feel like you are trapped in a relationship that is not working and you just want to feel special again, you want to feel alive! This is spiritual sickness.

Maybe it is not marriage but relationships in general. You just don't seem to fit in. Other people just seem so free and happy being in a crowd. Other people just seem so "with it" and seem to know their place in the world. But you just don't feel like you have anything in common with anyone, that you don't have a crowd to be with or a place to go. You might even be living a life in sexual sin feeling that this was the only thing that makes you feel good and the only thing you know. But you also know that you feel more distant than ever from other people and that you feel less and less accepted. This is spiritual sickness.

Maybe you just feel so worn down and useless. Maybe you are struggling with depression. You used to feel so young, alive, and attractive. Now, you just feel like another number, nothing special. You feel like you just want to be free and alive again. You want to feel confident again; you want to feel special and valuable. That is a spiritual sickness.

Maybe you are suffering from financial troubles. No matter what you do, there is just never enough money. You try to tuck away money. But every time you get a little money in the bank, something breaks like the air—conditioner or the car. It just feels like you're fighting an uphill battle. And on top of this, your spouse is never any help. All they want to do is spend money on what they want, never thinking about the future. You wonder where the money is going to come from if something really bad happens. You worry about paying the bills. What if I can't provide or protect the family. It just feels out of control and insecure . . . spiritual sickness.

Maybe, you are suffering from a lack of significance. You keep an active life, always going to sports games, movies, shows, parks. You are constantly hanging out with your friends and having fun. Or maybe it's the opposite—you never go out and just sit at home watching movies or TV. But busy or not, you can't seem to shake this sense that something is missing. It doesn't matter what you do, there is this part of you that feels like it is all in vain . . . illness of the spirit.

And maybe you are having a problem letting go. Maybe it is alcohol or drugs. You took a drink or the drug in high school or college out of interest but discovered that you are not strong enough to stop. Now it just feels like you'll never be free . . . spiritual illness.

Maybe you are having trouble letting go of anger or hurt. Someone said or did something to you or against you that you just can't seem to let go. You try to forgive, but how can you forgive something like that? That would be like saying "It's OK" and it's *not* OK! I know it is eating me up and hurting those around me; but I just can't let it go! . . . spiritual sickness.

Maybe you have a secret addiction, and you've been hiding the fact that you feel naked and afraid without it. Maybe you can see how it is wrecking your life around you but you don't know how to stop . . . spiritual illness.

Maybe you are into pornography and ashamed of it. It started with something as simple as your friend pulling out his dad's magazines and pointing out the girls in the bikinis. But then you found the wonderful world of the Internet. For women, it is the world of "erotic novels." But something has been happening. Your spouse has begun to seem less appealing. You can't stop gazing at the opposite sex without lustful thoughts, wondering what they look like without clothes, or looking forward to those times by yourself where you can gaze lustfully at those pictures or read those books . . . this is a deep spiritual illness.

***

The Doctor

Marriages on the brink of divorce, unruly and ungrateful kids, alcoholics, sexual addictions . . . etc. We have a sick society. And like all illnesses, we need someone who has the cure. And there is one who came a long time ago to be that cure who told us that he did not come to heal the healthy but the sick (Matthew 9:12). And he didn't come with a set of rules to teach us. He came because the problem is not with our physical self, our spiritual heart is sick.

And like all illnesses, if you go to the source and cure it from there, the whole body is cured. If you go to the source, you can stop the problem where it starts. On the other hand, if you try to put a Band-Aid on a gaping wound, it is not really going to help, the wound is likely to get worse, and the whole body might die. Listen to what this spiritual doctor said about this around 2,000 years ago:

"I am the vine; you are the branches. If a man remains in me and I in him, he will bear much fruit; apart from me you can do nothing. If anyone does not remain in me, he is like a branch that is thrown away and withers; such branches are picked up, thrown into the fire and burned. If you remain in me and my word remains in you, ask whatever you want and I will give it to you. This is my Father's glory, that you bear much fruit, showing yourselves to be my disciples."

My friends, we are all sick in some area of our lives because we are far from our source spiritually and we are not in relationship with God. We suffer because we don't know the truth and our lives are just the poor fruit from the withering tree. We don't know about our Father and Creator in Heaven. We don't know why we're created. And we definitely don't know how to be spiritually healthy.

**

Finding Spiritual Health and Joy

So how do you gain a relationship with your creator? Well, I'll tell you what you don't have to do. You don't have to go to church to get it. You also don't have to say a prayer over and over again repetitiously. You don't even have to give money. (Whew!) Since mankind is separated from God, out of his love for us, God gave us a pathway to reconciliation with him in the person of his son, Jesus the Christ. So the only thing you do have to do is to do what everyone does when they begin a relationship. You need to reach out and make contact. You need to talk to God and listen when he talks back. Then, you need to make a few simple statements and commit to relying on the truth of these statements. What you need to do is (paraphrased) to confess with your mouth and your heart that you want Jesus to be the Lord of your life and that you are choosing to believe in your heart that he was raised from the dead. When you do this you will be saved. (Romans 10:9). That's it. No tricks, no money exchanging hands, and no hoops to jump through; just say it and commit to it and your life can be forever changed.

Now, as someone who came kicking and screaming to the truth in Christ, I can only imagine the reactions to that last phrase. If you are like me, you are saying, "What, are you to tell me that by just saying that I believe in this person Jesus, that all my problems will go away?" Absolutely not; your problems will not go away. However, there are a few things that we are promised that make our problems bearable. I think Paul gave a great beginning list of just some of the things he called "the fruits of the spirit", meaning the benefits of putting God first. These fruits are love, joy, peace, patience, kindness, faithfulness, gentleness, and self-control. That doesn't sound too bad. And that is just in this life. We also get to live under the knowledge that we will be spending the rest of eternity in Heaven, free from all the pain and strife and in full relationship with God, our Father who loves us.

Remember what King Solomon said about the plant that is growing by the river. That will be you. You will be like "a tree planted by streams of water, which yields its fruit in season and whose leaf does not wither. Whatever [you] do prospers." You will know that God is working in your life because you will begin to see the fruit in your life. As good healthy trees produce good fruits and bad unhealthy trees produce bad fruits, so your life will be the same. If you make this decision to trust in Jesus and put your faith in Him, it will happen. Again, it doesn't mean that you won't have struggles and it won't mean that you are free from fear or doubt. But God tells us that "all work together for good, for those who are called according to His purpose." (Romans 8:28) Whatever happens in your life, if you just have faith and wait, you will see that God makes good out of it.

For some, these fruits can appear immediately. For others it might take a little while. But for those who truly believe and give their lives over to God, it does happen. So if you make this commitment and don't notice any changes in a month, don't doubt the truth. Go back to the beginning and ask yourself "do I really believe?" There is the beginning of salvation, in our belief.

When I confessed this prayer ten years ago, I was at the end of my rope. I was broke, we were on the verge of losing our home to the bank, my marriage was becoming dull and lifeless, I never had any joy in life, and the pressure kept multiplying to hold up my "house of cards". When Jesus opened my eyes enough to make the decision to follow Him and to allow Him to be the Lord of my life, it wasn't because I really wanted to nor that it even made sense to me. The whole idea seemed farfetched and ludicrous. But I decided to believe because nothing else in my life had worked until then. Even being a religion major and studying all kinds of world religions didn't make me feel any more knowledgeable or fulfilled. Today, I know that there is a lot of proof, not only that Jesus was alive, but that he was who he said he was. But back then, I ended up making the decision to trust in Jesus before I understood why or had any proof. But it was only when I gave my life to Jesus that I discovered who I was, why I was here, and what my purpose is. And it was only then that I first felt true joy.

***

Man Fully Alive

That that is my wish for you, that your eyes will be opened to who you really are; that you were created by God in heaven; that He knew you before even the beginnings of the world; that he has a plan for you and your life and that you will feel fulfilled and joyful every day knowing that you are on your path and that you are worthy and loved. St. Iraneus wrote a long time ago, "The glory of God is man fully alive." Would you like to be fully alive? Then make the choice and trust in Jesus. And for those who have eyes to see and ears to hear, just wait and see what He does in your life. I wish you the best and pray many blessings on you!

About the Author

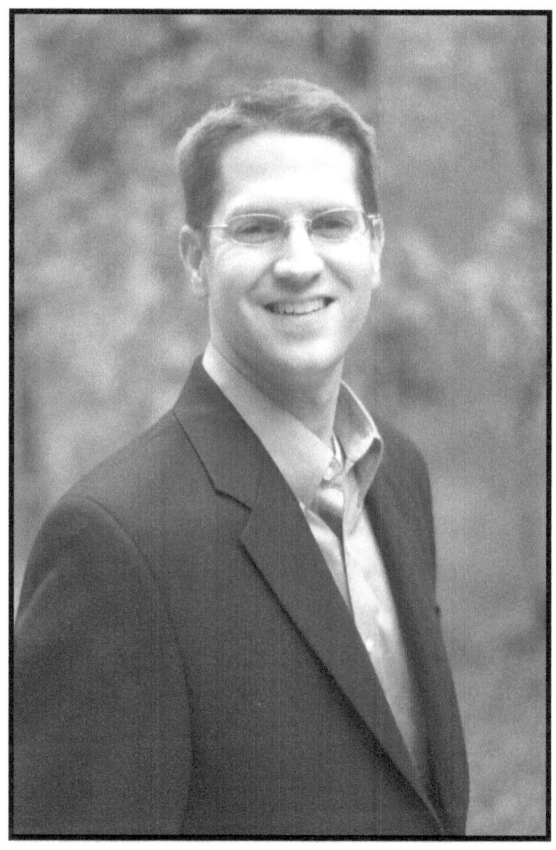

Tony Gonzalez is a freelance writer, a veteran of the United States Air Force, and a hypoglycemic. He has been studying diet and how it affects health for the last ten years and has made his own home a sugar-free zone. Tony is passionate about helping others, with the goal of helping them live happier and more productive lives. Tony lives in the suburbs of Atlanta, GA, with this wife and four children.

Index